Thanks for choosing this book. I wish you a good read and, if you like, leave a short review on Amazon. Thank you

Amy

SIRTFOOD DIET RECIPES

130+ Healthy Recipes Easy to Follow.
A Quick Start Guide to Promote Weight Loss, Detox,
and Antiaging Effect

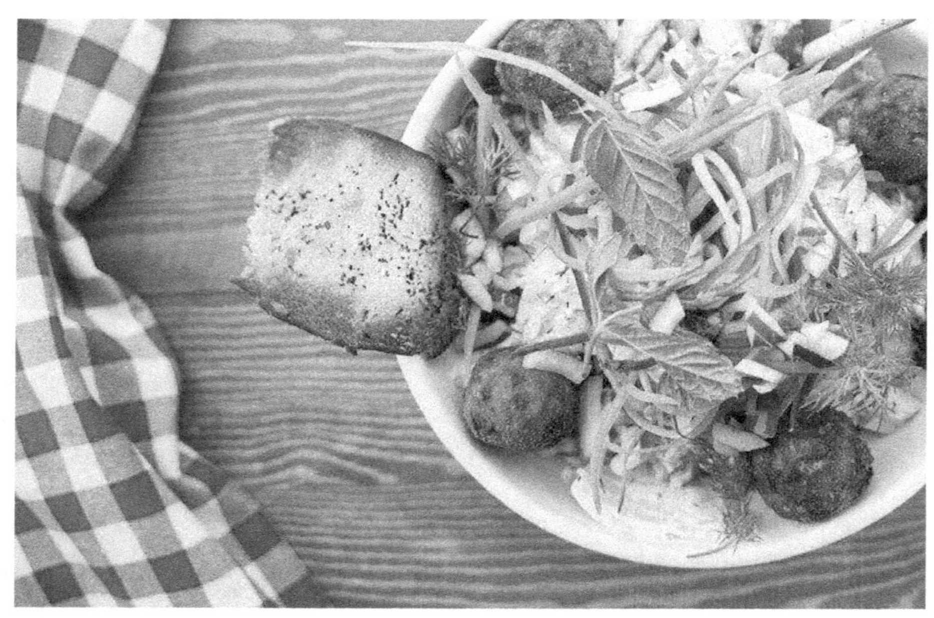

Amy Cook

Contents

Conclusion 179

Introduction

The consumption of sirtfood activates your body's natural fat-burning powers. Sirtuins control biological pathways, metabolism, lifespan, and cell function and are referred to as 'housekeeping genes.' Sirt foods are typically high in polyphenols and other antioxidants that activate your body's sirtuins. You'll burn more calories and revive your metabolism by including them in your diet. Research suggests that sirtuin activators control the production of insulin, enhance mitochondrial function, and boost lifespan.

The Sirtfood diet stresses eating foods that may interfere with a diet protein family known as sirtuin proteins. Sirtuins have been extensively researched, and preliminary studies have shown some promising effects. The Sirtfood diet is based on the idea that certain foods in your body cause sirtuins, which are particular proteins, believed to reap various benefits, from shielding cells in your body from inflammation to reversing aging.

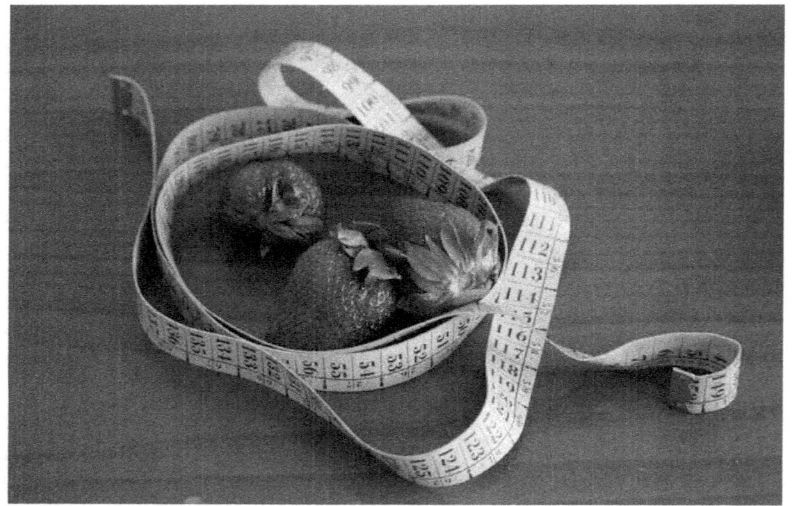

The Sirtfood Diet provides you with a fast, safe way to eat for weight loss, delicious easy-to-make recipes, and a long-term success maintenance plan. The Sirtfood Diet is a non-exclusion available and choices, and due to their antioxidant or anti-inflammatory effects, they can even provide some health benefits. Through sirtuin family member plays an integral role in controlling issues such as our metabolism, inner body clock, longevity, and aging.

Some researchers are calling sirtuins "skinny genes" for their potential role in weight loss because of the role they play in metabolism. There is growing evidence that activators of a sirtuin can have a wide range of health benefits, as well as muscle building and suppression of appetite.

These include helping the body in regulation of the levels of sugar in the blood, enhancing memory, and removing the damage done by free radical substances that accumulate in cells that causes cancer and other conditions.

There is strong observational evidence for the beneficial effects of food and drink consumption, rich in sirtuin activators, in reducing chronic disease risks. A Sirtfood diet is especially suited as an antiaging regime. While throughout the plant inclusion diet, and affordable. Sirtfoods are all readily potent activators of sirtuins.

Sirtuin Rich foods include certain fruits and vegetables, green tea, cocoa powder, and turmeric for the Indian spice, spinach, onions, and parsley. Many of the fruits and vegetables on sale in supermarkets, such as tomatoes, avocados, bananas, broccoli, kiwis, cabbage, and cucumber, are reportedly very small inactivators of sirtuin.

Nonetheless, this doesn't mean they aren't worth eating as they provide plenty of other advantages. The beauty of eating a sirtfood packed diet is that it's much more versatile than other foods. Simply adding some sirtfoods on top, you might eat healthily. Or you could be focused on getting them. A surprising result from one diet trial with Sirtfood is that participants lost substantial weight without losing muscle.

The increasing muscle was healthy for participants, leading to a more refined and toned look. That's the beauty of sirtfoods; it causes fat burning, but it also promotes maintenance, muscle growth, and repair. It is in complete contrast to many other diets where fat and muscle typically result in weight loss, with muscle loss slowing down the metabolism and making it more likely to lose weight.

You will find a variety of recipes that explore how you can tastefully and creatively work around the sirt ingredients and further enjoy the benefits it brings. All recipes you will find are typically good for one serving or two, and most recipes that are beyond the serving of 2 are those recipes that you can snack on or store in the refrigerator or freezer so for you have ready to grab food during those days where your schedule might be hectic.

Before we go further into our recipes, the 1st part will tell us more about the sirtuins and more on the benefits of each ingredient. For the 2nd part, it will be purely recipes divided into types of meals and types of meat used. Hipe, you enjoy learning and discovering what might become your new favorite recipe.

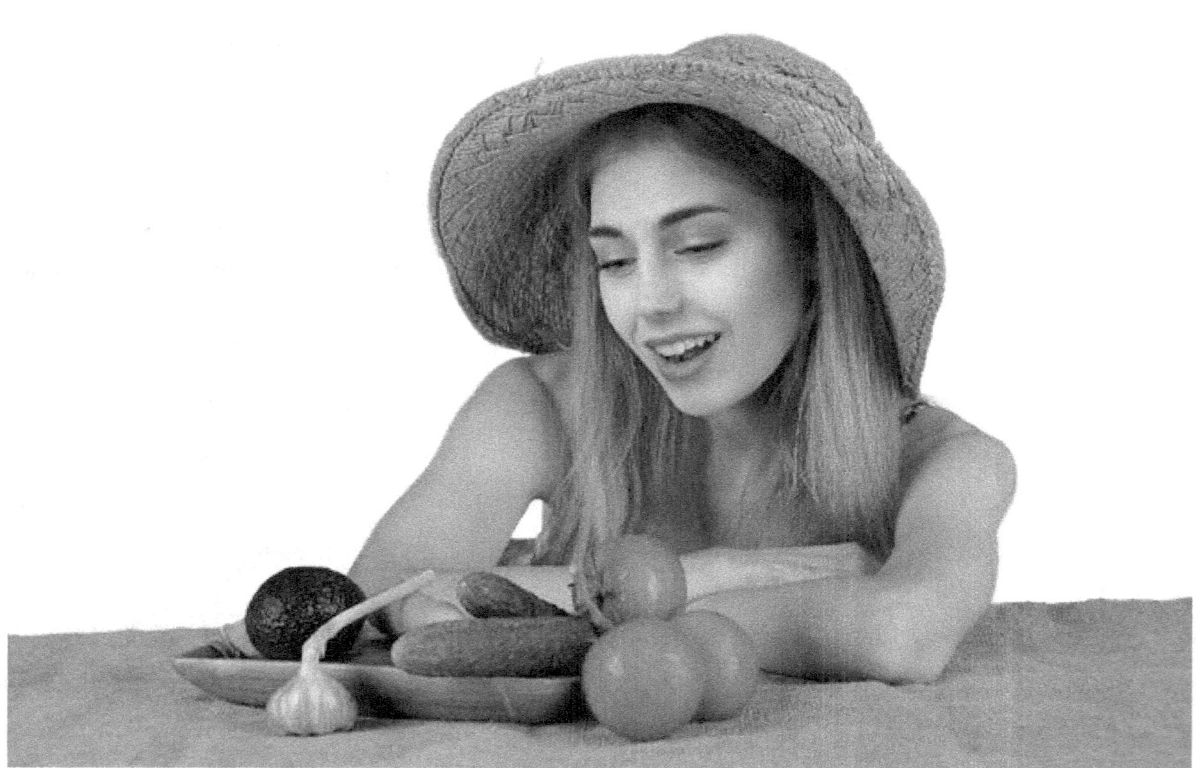

Chapter 1

What are Sirtuins?

Sirtuins are for metabolic function, and it is a delicate combination of consumption, usage, and conservation of energy. Sirtuins are the nicotinamide adenine dinucleotide (NAD+) family of dependent deacetylases.

They are found to be critical sensors in the MTN, controlling energy homeostasis, lipid balance, and glucose metabolism as a reaction to physiological changes in energy rates. Sirtuins not only modulate cytoplasmic and mitochondria proteins, deacetylated histones, and other transcriptional regulators in the nucleus. Not too long ago, as the Holy Grail, sirtuins acquired considerable nutriceutical value to prolong their lifespan.

The work was carried out to classify activators of this young spring, and resveratrol, the most potent sirtuin activator, became the family name for polyphenol are present in red wine, berries, and peanuts. That was another legitimate excuse for consuming red wine when you were toasting for a long time. Although, not yet entirely transferable to humans, sirtuins have been connected to survival in yeasts, worms, flies, and mice.

One or two Sirtuins can promote mitochondria function. The cell's powerhouses and mitochondrial proteins play a significant role in metabolism-related diseases such as type 2 diabetes and obesity, but it is also a neurodegressive disease.

Much remains to be understood before a modern Ponce de Leon can claim this exact sirtuin activation function. In the meantime, you should also toast to good health, as sirtuins play a significant role in proper metabolic maintenance.

In mammals, seven proteins (SIRT1–SIRT7) in the sirtuin family are distinct in terms of tissue specificity, sub-cellular position, and enzyme activity, and target. The following grades are class I (SIRT1–SIRT3), class II (SIRT4), class III (SIRT5), and class IV (SIRT6 and SIRT7).

They are into four groups' classification. Sirtuins have recently been identified as ADP-ribosyl transferases, in addition to their original function as histone deacetylases, and also have demalonymisation and desuccinylation activity with a broad range of target protein.

Sirtuin
•SIRT1
•SIRT2
•SIRT3
•SIRT4
•SIRT5
•SIRT6
•SIRT7

SIRT1, the better-described sirtuin, has been researched for its function in lowering calories, avoiding aging-related diseases, and maintaining metabolic homeostasis. In low nutrition environments, such as hunger, SIRT1 expression is upregulated and repressed with surplus sugar, such as a high-fat diet.

SIRT1 prevents adipogenesis and enhances fat mobilization through lipolysis in the differentiated adipocyte cell lines. SIRT1 promotes the mounting of an NCor1 and SMRT co-repressor complex to PPARα target gene promoters for repressing their transcription, thus restricting fat storage in caloric and fasting situations.

SIRT1 deacetylation of PPARα co-activator (PGC1α) is a transcript co-regulator that regulates biogenesis and development in mitochondria. It contributes to the activation of PGC1α as well as induction of pathways downstream that regulate mitochondrial gene expression.

SIRT1 also regulates the acetylation in transcription factors of forkhead box O (FOXO), which is essential lipid and glucose metabolism regulators, as well as stress responses.

FOXO's deacetylation mediated by SIRT1 was proposed to direct FOXO to its selective goals.

In metabolic homeostasis, SIRT2 may play a function of deacetylating carboxykinase of phosphoenolpyruvate, which is the kinase that includes gluconeogenesis and inhibits its degradation through ubiquitination. SIRT2 also deacetylates and stimulates the Adipogenesis FOXO1.

SIRT3 is the major mitochondrial deacetylase, located mainly in mitochondria. Many of its goals play a significant role in metabolic homeostasis.

Long-chain acyl CoA dehydrogenase (LCAD)

This is a fatty oxidation enzyme that has long-fasting SIRT3, which aims to inhibit LCAD hyperacetylation and fatty acid degradation. Removing SIRT3 in mice impairs fat degradation, increases dietary obesity, and reduces cold-exposure immunity during fasting. In 3-hydroxy-3-methylglutaryl CoA synthase 2, which governs the development of ketone bodies, which is an essential source of energy for the brain while blood glucose levels are small.

SIRT3 deacetylation sites have also been established. In response to caloric restrictions, SIRT3 isocitrate dehydrogenase 2 deacetylates/activates is involved in the Krebs cycle and the GDH cancer cycle enzyme. SIRT3 also deacetylates the pathway components of mitochondrial aerobic breathing.

SIRT4 acts by ADP-ribosylating GDH in metabolism, inhibiting its function and blocking amino acid secretion. SIRT4 also controls the oxidation of hepatocytes and myocytes by fatty acids. Short RNA hairpin-mediated SIRT4 liver knockdown increases oxidative fatty acid. SIRT3 and SIRT4 tend to have different functions in GDH control and fatty acid oxidation.

SIRT5 targets carbamoyl phosphate synthetase 1, whose deacetylation activates ammonia detoxification by the urea cycle during fasting.

SIRT6 not only plays a part in the maintenance and regeneration of DNA but also in metabolism and aging. SIRT6−/− Mice die in early adulthood, have reduced insulin growth factor (IGF) 1 and are highly hypoglycemic, with adverse muscle and brown adipose glucose absorption. Specifically, blazing SIRT6 in birth mice leads to lower body weight (due to reduced levels of the IGF1), which normalizes at the age of 1 year, but then, later on, develops into obesity.

Although it is understood that SIRT7 stimulates transcription of RNA polymerase 1, its protein substratum is still unclear.

The Science of Sirtuins

Sirtuins allow the cellular wellbeing to be controlled. You have to understand how it functions, what it can do with the body, and why it relies on NAD+ to function.

Sirtuins are a class of cell safety controlling proteins. Sirtuins play a crucial function in cell homeostasis control. Homeostasis requires equilibrium of the organism. However, only NAD+, nicotinamide adenine dinucleotide, and coenzyme found in all the living cells are capable of functioning in sirtuins.

How Sirtuins Regulate Cellular Health with NAD+

Think of the cells of your body like an office. Many employees operate on various duties in the workplace with the same purpose: remain competitive and accomplish the company's goal as effectively as possible. There are numerous parts in the cells that work on several tasks with the ultimate objective, too: stay healthy and function as long as possible efficiently.

Just as company priorities change because of different internal and external factors, so are cell priorities. Someone should run the office and regulate what happens when who will do it and when to change course. That will be the CEO in the workplace. It's your sirtuins in the body, on the cellular level.

Sirtuins are a seven-protein family that plays an essential role in cell safety. Only NAD+, nicotinamide adenine dinucleotide, a coenzyme found in all living cells, may function as sirtuins. NAD+ is essential for the metabolism of cells and hundreds of other biological processes.

When sirtuins become the CEO of a business, then NAD+ is the money that covers the CEO 's salaries and employees when keeping the lights on and paying office rent. Without it, a company and the body cannot work. But NAD+ levels decrease with age, limiting sirtuins' function with age. It's not that easy, like other stuff in the human body.

Sirtuins manage all that takes place in your cells.

Sirtuins are a protein family. Protein may sound like dietary protection — as found in bovine and meat, and protein shakes, well — but we're talking here of protein molecules that work in several functions throughout the body's cells. You can think of proteins as divisions in an organization, each of which works on its unique task in collaboration with other divisions.

Hemoglobin is a recognized protein in the body that is part of the globin protein family, which is essential for the distribution of oxygen in the blood. Myoglobin is the equivalent of the hemoglobin, and together they make up the globin family.

The body has nearly 60,000 protein families — with several divisions! — And one of those families is sirtuins. Although hemoglobin is one of a two-protein band, sirtuins are seven in a band.

There are three of the seven sirtuins in the cell working in mitochondria, three in the core, and one in the cytoplasm playing several roles. However, the essential function of sirtuins is to extract acetyl groups from specific proteins.

Acetyl groups regulate similar reactions. These are actual protein tags that other proteins known can respond to. When proteins are the cell divisions, and DNA is the Chairman, the acetyl community is increasing the department head's availability status. For starters, if a protein is present, the sirtuin will interact with it to do anything like the CEO can function with a department manager.

Sirtuins function with acetyl groups by what is known as deacetylation. This implies that an acetyl group is recognized on a molecule. The acetyl group extracts the molecule for its function. One way sirtuins function is to detach biological proteins such as histones from acetyl groups (deacetylating).

Sirtuins, for example, are deacetylated histones, proteins in a condensed form of DNA known as chromatin. The histone is a big voluminous protein which is wound around the DNA. Call it a Christmas tree, and the DNA beach is the main cove. The chromatin is free or unwound when the histones have an acetyl ring.

The unwound chromatin ensures that the DNA, a crucial organ, is transcribed. However, it doesn't have to stay unwound, as it is vulnerable to injury, just like the Christmas lights will tangle themselves, or the bulbs can get broken, whether they are too rough or too big. As sirtuins deacetylate the histones, the chromatin is closed, or the gene expression ceases or silences firmly and neatly.

For about 20 years we have only known sirtuins, and their primary function was found in the 1990s. Since then, scholars have flocked to study them and established their significance and posed concerns about what else we could know.

The Discovery and History of Sirtuins

The first sirtuin, called SIR2, was discovered by Dr. Amar Klar in the 1970s as a gene that controls the capacity of leaven cells to mate. Years later, in the 1990s, researchers identified specific genes that were — identical in form — homologous to SIR2 in certain species such as mice, fruit flies, also called sirtuins. Each organism had different numbers of sirtuins. For starters, yeast has five sirtuins, one has bacteria, seven have mice, and seven have humans.

In 1991, along with Nick Austriaco and Brian Kennedy, Elysium's co-founder and MIT scientist Leonard Guarente performed research on how yeast was aging. Luckily, Austriaco tried to grow yeast crops from samples that he had been storing for months in his fridge that produced a stressful environment for the strains.

Many of the strains could only develop from here, but Guarente and his team established a pattern: the yeast strains which lasted the best in the refrigerator were also the most extended living. This led Guarente to focus solely on these long-lived strains of yeast.

This contributed to SIR2 being identified as a gene that facilitated yeast survival. It is important to note that there is no evidence to date that this study can be extrapolated to humans, and further research on the effects of SIR2 on humans is necessary.

The Guarente lab, therefore, observed that eliminating SIR2 shortened leaven life significantly, although growing the number of copies of the SIR2 gene from one to two, increased the yeast life period. Yet, of course, what triggered SIR2 has yet to be identified.

This is where groups of acetyl come into play. At first, it was believed that SIR2 could be an enzyme deacetylating — which indicates that certain acetyl groups were separated — from other molecules. Still, no one understood if that was valid, as all attempts to demonstrate that behavior in a test tube proved negatively.

Guarente and his colleagues observed that in the presence of NAD+, nicotinamide adenine dinucleotide, SIR2 in yeast could only deacetylate specific proteins.

Chapter 2

Scientific Evidence of Sirtuins

Sirtuins are a group of proteins that manage cell wellbeing. Sirtuins assume a crucial job in controlling cell homeostasis.

In the workplace, numerous individuals are taking a shot at different assignments with an ultimate objective: remain gainful and productively satisfy the strategic the organization for whatever length of time that conceivable.

In the cells, numerous pieces are taking a shot at different undertakings with a final objective, as well: remain sound and capacity proficiently for whatever length of time that conceivable. Similarly, as needs in the organization change, because of different inside and outer variables, so do needs in the cells. Somebody needs to run the workplace, directing what completes when, who will do it and when to switch course.

NAD+ is essential to cell digestion and many other organic procedures. If sirtuins are an organization's CEO, at that point, NAD+ is the cash that pays the pay of the CEO and workers, all while keeping the lights on and the workplace space lease paid. An organization, and the body, can't work without it.

Protein may seem like dietary protein — what's found in beans and meats and well, protein shakes — yet for this situation, we're discussing atoms called proteins, which work all through the body's phones in various capacities. Consider proteins the divisions at an organization, everyone concentrating without anyone else explicit capacity while planning with different offices.

Acetyl bunches control explicit responses. They're physical labels on proteins that different proteins perceive will respond with them. In the event that proteins are the branches of the cell, and DNA is the CEO, the acetyl bunches are the accessibility status of every division head.

For instance, in the event that a protein is accessible, at that point, the sirtuin can work with it to get something going, similarly as the CEO can work with an available division head to get something going.

Sirtuins work with acetyl bunches by doing what's called deacetylation. One way that sirtuins work is by evacuating acetyl gatherings deacetylating organic proteins, for example, histones. The histone is an enormous cumbersome protein that the DNA folds itself over.
This loosened up chromatin implies the DNA is being translated, a fundamental procedure.

We've just thought about sirtuins for around 20 years, and their essential capacity was found during the 1990s. From that point forward, specialists have rushed to examine them, recognizing their significance while likewise bringing up issues about what else we can find out about them.

In 1991, Elysium fellow benefactor and MIT scientist Leonard Guarente, close by graduate understudies Nick Austriaco and Brian Kennedy, directed tests to all the more likely see how yeast matured. By some coincidence, Austriaco attempted to develop societies of different yeast strains from tests he had put away in his ice chest for quite a long time, which made an unpleasant situation for the strains.

This is the place acetyl bunches become possibly the most essential factor. It was at the first idea that SIR2 may be a deacetylating protein — which means it expelled those acetyl gatherings — from different atoms, however, nobody knew whether this was valid since all endeavors to show this movement in a test tube demonstrated negative.
In Guarente's very own words: "Without NAD+, SIR2 sits idle. That was the basic finding on the circular segment of sirtuin science."

Ecological factors significantly influence the destiny of living beings, and sustenance is one of the most persuasive variables. These days life span is a significant objective of medicinal science and has consistently been a fabrication for the individual since antiquated occasions. Precisely, endeavors are planned for accomplishing effective maturing, to be specific a long life without genuine ailments, with a decent degree of physical and mental autonomy and satisfactory social connections.

Gathering information unmistakably exhibits that it is conceivable to impact the indications of maturing. Without a doubt, wholesome mediations can advance wellbeing and life span. A tribute must be given to Ancel Keys, who was the first to give definite logical proof about the job of sustenance in the wellbeing/sickness balance at the populace level, explicitly in connection to cardiovascular illness, still the primary source of death overall.

It is commonly valued that the sort of diet can significantly impact the quality and amount of life, and the Mediterranean eating regimen is paradigmatic of an advantageous dietary example. The developing cognizance of the beneficial impacts of a particular dietary example on wellbeing and life span in the other 50% of the only remaining century produced a ground-breaking push toward structuring eats fewer carbs that could diminish the danger of constant maladies, subsequently bringing about solid maturing.

Subsequently, during the 1990s, the Dietary Approaches to Stop Hypertension Dash diet was contrived so as to assess whether it was conceivable to treat hypertension, not pharmacologically. To be sure, the DASH diet was very like the Mediterranean Diet, being wealthy in foods grown from the ground, entire grains, and strands, while deficient in creature soaked fats and cholesterol.

The excellent news leaving the investigation was that not exclusively did the DASH diet lower circulatory strain. However, it additionally diminished the danger of cardiovascular infection, type 2 diabetes, a few sorts of malignant growth. Other maturing related maladies To additionally improve the medical advantages of plant nourishment prosperous, creature fat-terrible eating routines, especially in hypercholesterolemic people, the Portfolio Diet was planned

This eating regimen, other than being to a great extent veggie-lover, with just limited quantities of saturated fats, prescribes a high admission of utilitarian nourishments, including thick filaments, plant stanols, soy proteins, and almonds likewise. Curiously, members on the Portfolio Diet displayed a decrease of coronary illness chance related to lower plasma cholesterol and incendiary files in contrast with members on a sound, for the most part, vegan diet.

Nonetheless, additionally, the measure of ingested nourishment has been pulling in light of a legitimate concern for mainstream researchers as a potential modifier of the harmony among wellbeing and infection in a wide range of living species. Individually, calorie limitation CR has been exhibited to be a rising healthful intercession that animates the counter maturing instruments in the body.

In this way, the eating routine of the individuals living on the Japanese island of Okinawa has been widely broken down on the grounds that these islanders are notable for their life span and expanded wellbeing range, bringing about the best recurrence of centenarians on the planet. Interestingly, the customary Okinawan diet came about to be fundamentally the same as the Mediterranean Diet and the DASH diet regarding nourishment types.

Be that as it may, the vitality admission of Okinawans, at the hour of the underlying logical perceptions, was about 20% lower than the standard vitality admission of the Japanese, along these lines deciding an average state of CR.

Singer Adele has confirmed that she has lost 30 kilos in just one year. The secret? Apparently, it's all thanks to the Sirtfood Diet. It was revealed by the singer herself through international media, such as the Daily Mail and the New York Post.

The Sirtfood Diet is not the classic fasting diet: Adele is the living proof of this, given the beautiful shape in which was at her appointments with her fans. It is, in fact, a diet that leaves room for both cheese and red wine as well as chocolate, in the right proportions, and of course under the supervision of a specialist doctor, who knows how to evaluate your health and recommend the most suitable diet to lose weight safely.

Many were the media that underlined the substantial weight loss of the singer Adele who admitted, how the decision to lose weight did not depend on the acceptance of herself as much as the difficulty of using her voice to the fullest.

Adele praised the Sirtfood Diet, which made her lose 30 kilos without much effort. In reality, she admitted via Instagram that she had never struggled as much in physical activity as when preparing for her tour). She also said that the beauty of Sirt foods is that many of them are already on our table every day. They are accessible and can be easily integrated into our diet.

Although being thinner was not her priority the singer has always had an excellent relationship with her body), she wanted to review her eating habits to get back in shape, but also or better above all to feel good about herself.

Furthermore, the Sirtfood Diet had come back on the news because it was Pippa Middleton's choice to get back into shape quickly before her wedding with the millionaire James Matthews that was celebrated on May 20, 2017.

Chapter 3

Advantages of Sirtuins

In our Sirtfood Diet, preliminary members lost a great 7 pounds over the underlying 7 days remembering increments for muscle and muscle work. This emotional impact on fat-consuming, while advancing muscle, is one reason that our Sirtfood-based diet has gotten so mainstream with anybody needing to get slender and fit as a fiddle, much the same as the world-class competitors and models.

They have supported along these lines of eating. Alongside fat consumption, Sirtfoods additionally have the extraordinary capacity to usually satisfy hunger, making them the ideal answer for accomplishing a healthy weight and continuing it long haul.

Be that as it may, to consider it absolutely as a weight loss diet is to overlook the main issue. This is a diet that has a lot to do with health as waistlines. Expanded vitality, brighter skin, feeling progressively alarmed, and better rest are the charming 'symptoms' from along these lines of eating.

Now and again, the advantages are much progressively exceptional, remembering situations where following the diet for the more drawn out term has turned around metabolic ailments. Such is their wellbeing improving impacts that reviews demonstrate them to be all the more dominant then physician endorsed medicates in forestalling constant malady, with benefits in diabetes, coronary illness, and Alzheimer's to give some examples.

It's no big surprise that it is entrenched that the way of life eating the most Sirtfoods has been the least fatty and most beneficial on the planet. The primary concern is clear: If you need to accomplish a progressively fiery, less fatty, and more advantageous body, and establish the frameworks for lifelong wellbeing and protection from sickness, then the Sirtfood Diet is for you.

Here at the International Food Information Council Foundation, we ramble about trend diets. For the most part, we're exposing them and advancing a fair eating arrangement with space for guilty pleasures and festivities. Now and then, the diets we talk about depending on some strong sustenance rules, and others we can't accept truly exist.

This next diet we're going to discuss falls into the last class. The most recent on the diet scene is the sirtfood diet, and we're here to disclose to you why you needn't bother with that sort of limitation in your life: It's not science-based or practical.

Here are three motivations to take a pass on the sirtfood diet:

The sirtfood diet estimates achievement is just as far as weight loss.
I've said it before, and I'll state it once more: Weight is a determinant of wellbeing, yet it's not alone. To gauge somebody's wellbeing accomplishment on whether they lose X pounds in X measure of time overlooks the various advantages of nourishment. Nourishment is brimming with vitality, which enables you to do things like showering, practicing, and relaxing.

It additionally has supplements that can advance a few substantial capacities and is often a cheerful encounter established in custom. For by and large wellbeing, there's a great deal more to concentrate on than basic appearance, and estimating achievement just as far as weight loss is incomprehensive.

It's prohibitive, which can harm your association with nourishment.
This diet stresses an admission of 1,000 to 1,500 calories every day, which is a lot of lower than a great many people need. When we seriously limit our nourishment admission, our intuitive response is to indulge. Your body is savvy, and it thinks about this absence of sustenance as an assault. Therefore, we will, in general, overcompensate, which is the reason we as a whole can identify with being "hangry" and like this overindulging when we're at last allowed to eat. Rehearsing careful and intuitive eating is a more practical course than confining nourishment.

The sirtfood diet isn't science-based.
While there is some questionable research about the advantages of sirtuins, there's practically zero research about the specific sirtfood diet. Moreover, we, as of now, have a few rules set up that have been completely looked into and tried for quite a long time. If you're lost on what "sound nourishment" is, this is a superior spot to begin.

It's thoroughly fine if you need to join a couple sirtfoods into an eating plan. Nourishments like green tea, organic product, dim chocolate, and kale all include a spot inside a smart dieting design! Be that as it may, holding fast to a program with such exacting pass-or-bomb prerequisites is unreasonable and could be hurtful to your association with nourishment.

By fusing an eating plan that is loaded with assortment and eating carefully, you'll have the option to set up a long haul, manageable association with nourishment. Cheers to that!

THE RISING INCIDENCE of corpulence related ailments, for example, diabetes, dyslipidemia, and cardiovascular and cerebrovascular sicknesses in industrialized nations, have become a general medical issue vital. Numerous helpful and preventive systems to forestall or battle corpulence have come around.

However, few have endured the trial of time. One marvel that got the enthusiasm for this setting is the alleged "French oddity." First noted by Irish doctor Samuel Black in 1819, the French Catch 22 makes an inference to the way that the French are seen as having a moderately low occurrence of cardiovascular and metabolic infection, even though their eating regimen is wealthy in immersed fat.

The high utilization of red wine, which is rich in the polyphenol resveratrol, is believed to be one of the essential elements adding to this particular preferred position.

In the interim, since the 1930s, it has been likewise notable that caloric limitation CR can hinder the maturing procedure and defer the beginning of various maturing related illnesses, for example, malignancy, cardiovascular infections, and metabolic ailments. CR altogether extends life expectancy in living beings running from yeast and nematodes to rodents and monkeys 1, 2).

Strikingly, the valuable wellbeing results of CR look like those that are prompted by resveratrol in various creature models, proposing that the atomic pathways by which resveratrol acts are like those initiated by CR.

As of late, it was proposed that the sirtuins could be the regular go-betweens that clarify both the impacts of resveratrol and CR pathways. In this survey, we will talk about the atomic system that underlies the organic action of these sirtuins, their useful jobs in entire body physiology, and their potential relationship to human maladies.

Chapter 4

The Discovery of the SirtFood Diet

The Sirt Diet was conceived and recently proposed by two British nutritionists, Aidan Goggins and Glen Matten, nutrition science professionals who have worked both in Ireland and in Great Britain, collaborating with the medical team of a highly rated London sports club, and have been involved in preparing the food program of well-known sports personalities, such as Olympic sailing champion Ben Ainslie, boxer Anthony Ogogo, as well as celebrities such as models Jodie Kidd and Lorraine Pascale and more recently the famous singer Adele who has depopulated on the web.

Even the sister of Duchess of Cambridge, Pippa Middleton, opt for this diet before her wedding day. The Sirt diet is based on scientific research and on a pilot project that has led to surprising results. Surprising because one can see the drastic changes without people getting unhealthy.

"Usually - as the nutritionists themselves explain - when you lose weight, you lose a little fat, but also muscle: it happens in practically every diet. If someone loses 3.2 kilos in a week on a normal diet, you can rest assured that at least 900 grams are of muscle. When we checked the effects of our diet, we were speechless: muscle mass not only had not decreased but had increased by an average of 900 grams ".

It was a very important discovery that helped to conclude and experience the profound effects of Sirt foods on metabolism. These foods not only activate the consumption of fats but also promote muscle growth and repair. "The more you have muscles - continue Goggins and Matten - the more you burn energy, even when you are at rest. With a normal diet instead, when you lose weight, you lose fat, and therefore, your metabolism slows down".

This is the main feature of this food plan that makes this diet an innovative path, different from all the diets you are used to thinking about. It has been talked about in the Anglo-Saxon newspapers for months now, especially after the photo that the English singer Adele has posted to thank the fans for the good wishes for her 32nd birthday has left many speechless.

We immediately thought about the intervention of a cosmetic surgeon. Still, behind the new image of the singer and other VIP characters, there is not this time the scalpel, but a diet, the Sirtfood Diet.

The term appeared for the first time in 2017 when the two researchers proposed it. Still, it was in 2019 that it reached popularity, so much so that, according to Google, it was one of the most sought after diets of last year and certainly one of the most mysterious and successful.

This nutritional program is characterized not only by the attention paid to the recruitment of what the two experts call Sirt Food but also by the calorie restriction. Only by combining these two points, according to Goggins and Matten, is it possible to lose weight.

Let's find out what it is and how it works.

Chapter 5

How Sirtfoods Help to Burn Fat

The most significant benefit of the sirtfood diet is its incredible impact on losing fats from the body. Fats are made up of fatty acids that combine to make adipocytes. These adipocytes are clusters of fatty acids, and unlike free fatty acids, adipocytes are not mostly present in the blood. They get accumulated under skin, in muscles, and on different organs.

These adipocytes combine to make adipose tissues, which are full fledge foam-shaped cluster of visible yellowish white-colored fat in our body. Adipocytes are the most healthy fat cells to burn. They must have been broken down into adipocytes and finally in free fatty acids (in reverse order of formation) to get burned from the fat-burning enzymes called the lipase enzyme.

These steps are not easy as they seem, and burning extra pounds of fats can be a hard nut to crack. The most challenging step in this cycle is to break adipose tissues in adipocytes. The sirtfoods contain high levels of polyphenols. To be very specific, sirtfoods are those which contain high levels of a chemical compound called polyphenol.

This compound is not uniformly distributed in sirtfoods, but every sirtfood contains specific amounts of polyphenols. Polyphenols are the compounds that are present naturally in sirtfood, and many types of research conducted on these foods have confirmed that these foods have the highest impacts when losing extra pounds of fats from the body.

Polyphenols are essential precursors in the fat burning cycle of the body called lipolysis. Free fatty acids in our blood are subjected to digestion and then excretion from the body through an enzyme called lipase.

Foods rich in Polyphenols cause much increase in levels of lipase enzyme and thus more fat burning blits in the body. Polyphenols act on lipase and other fat-burning mediators by activating a particular type of gene in the body called sirtuin.

This gene is the most crucial part of the sirtfood diet because, through this gene activation, polyphenol-rich foods called the sirtfoods act on extra stored fat in our body and engine a fat-burning cycle in our body to get rid of it. Sirtuin gene is a human gene and present in every human.

The fuel of the body is glucose, which is the most readily available nutrient in the body for energy. The glucose is broken down into energy packets called ATPs, which are produced from the power of cells called mitochondria. These energy packets are utilized to fuel the body while performing actions.

High-intensity work such as exercise requires a much more significant amount of energy as compared to typing on a keyboard. The higher the intensity of work, the larger will be the needed amount of ATPs. The most significant source of glucose in the body is carbohydrates, which are sugars in simpler forms. A diet rich in low glycemic carbohydrates is essential while performing high-intensity tasks.

These carbohydrates are broken down into the purest form of sugar called glucose. This glucose undergoes a series of reactions called the glycolysis. In this cycle, the end product is the ATPs that are stored or utilized in response to stress produced in the body. These ATPs are also crucial for fighting against the infections because the higher the level of energy in the body, the greater will be the immune response of the body.

All the processes are directly proportional. When the body is stimulated through the intake of foods containing this protein called "super metabolic regulator," the so-called "lean gene" is activated which allows you to burn energy by reproducing the same effects of fasting and physical activity (it makes you lose weight, increases muscle mass and improves the general condition of the organism).

The sirtfood diet is affluent in proteins, good fats, and low glycemic carbohydrates. All these macronutrients are essential for fulfilling the body's essential needs of energy and refueling.

Let's get to the practice: how does it work? The Sirt diet involves a first phase divided into two parts. The first, which lasts 3 days, prescribes the intake of a maximum of 1,000 Calories in the form of 3 vegetable juices and a solid meal based on Sirt foods. The second phase (from day 4 to day 7) brings the maximum calorie intake to 1,500 calories. It involves the consumption of 2 vegetable juices and 2 solid meals based on Sirt foods.

The second phase corresponds to what is generally called "maintenance," lasts 14 days, and involves the consumption of 1 vegetable juice and 3 balanced meals rich in Sirt foods.

According to the promises of Goggins and Matten in the first week, you should lose about 3.2 kg. Even in the maintenance phase, you may lose weight, but it is not its main goal. How to lose more weight? In fact, according to the two nutritionists, you could repeat the diet as many times as you want.

The fundamental rule of the Sirt diet is therefore always to include the so-called Sirt foods in daily meals, which, according to the two creators, would help the body burn the calories more easily and quickly, thus promoting rapid weight loss without too many sacrifices.

Looking at the results achieved by Adele, it seems that yes, the Sirt diet works. As always, however, you should not only worry about how many pounds you can lose but also what you are going to burn. As with all diets, even in this case, you must dispose of excess fat without affecting the muscles.

Goggins and Matten ensure that the Sirt diet does not lead to a loss of muscle mass. They also claim that you would not run the risk of regaining weight after the diet and that you would avoid both increasing physical activity to lose weight and suffering from hunger.

However, if you dwell on its functioning, you can easily notice how in the first phase, it is, in fact, a low-calorie diet and how the allowed calories are very few.

There is, therefore, some doubt as to whether the rapid initial weight loss may be due at least in part to a loss of glycogen (the body's supply of glucose) and water instead of fat; only if official data are published that show that most of those lost pounds correspond to fat can you be sure that the Sirt diet can guarantee what it promises you.

For the rest, information on the benefits associated with the activation of the Sirt genes is not lacking. The foods whose consumption is encouraged are ingredients that are widespread in food regimes with proven health benefits, such as our Mediterranean diet. My advice is to have a nutritionist follow you even if you decide to follow the Sirt diet. This way, you will avoid taking risks when you decide to reduce your food intake as much as is foreseen in the first phase.

I also recommend that you do not underestimate the benefits of combining diet and physical activity. If you get into the habit of exercising regularly, it will be easier for you to avoid losing weight.

Chapter 6

Sirtuin Staples

Buckwheat

Many people do not include buckwheat into their daily diets, but you should. Not only is it a great source of fiber, but it is also high in protein, and the carbohydrates will energize you when your calorie intake is limited.

By adding in some buckwheat to your meals, you will help them stick with you longer, keeping you satisfied and energized longer than you otherwise would be. Another great bonus of buckwheat is that it is gluten-free, making it perfect for people with gluten intolerance or Celiac disease. Buckwheat is a grain, or rather a pseudocereal, that is great for heart health.

Dark Chocolate/Cocoa

A diet that allows chocolate? Yes! However, you can't mindlessly eat any variety or endless amounts of chocolate. While chocolate may be a great sirtfood, it's high in calories, meaning that excessive servings can interfere with weight loss.

Thankfully, since the Sirt diet manages calorie control, you shouldn't eat too much if you follow the guidelines. You should also stick with cocoa or dark chocolate 70% or higher. While milk and white chocolate may be delicious, they do not have the same health benefits.

One of the biggest benefits of dark chocolate is the role it plays in heart health. As many of the antioxidant sirtuins found within it are varieties especially helpful for heart health, you will find you can greatly reduce your risk of cardiovascular disease.

Coffee

You may only think of coffee as a necessity to stay awake, or worse; you might even consider it an unhealthy addiction. However, just like tea has health benefits, so too makes coffee. In a single cup of coffee, you can get plenty of vitamins B2, B3, B5, potassium, and manganese.

Medjool Dates

Grown in the tropics, most of the dates you find in Western countries are the dried variety. They are highly sweet and chewy and are sometimes even sold in the form of date sugar to be used in baked goods, coffee, or anything else you might want to sweeten. This is beneficial, as coconut palm sugar has more health benefits than cane sugar. However, keep in mind that it is still a form of sugar and should only be enjoyed in moderation.

Kale

Kale is categorized as a calciferous vegetable, is a member of the cabbage family, and is considered one of the most nutritionally-dense foods on earth. A single cup serving of ale contains large numbers of vitamins K, A, C, and B6, along with the minerals manganese, copper, calcium, magnesium, and potassium. All of this nutrition is packed in only thirty-three calories, making it a great choice to add to your daily diet.

Rocket Arugula

Arugula is unlike many other forms of lettuce, as it has a much stronger flavor that is distinct and peppery, adding a delicious flavor to a number of dishes. Even if a dish doesn't call for arugula, you can frequently add it in addition to or instead of other types of lettuce. Arugula is rich in potassium, calcium, vitamin C, vitamin K, vitamin A, and folate.

The calcium and vitamin K found in arugula are both critical for proper bone health. We are taught the value of calcium all through childhood. But, many people are unaware of the role that is played by vitamin K. Simply put, if you want healthy bones, then you must consume enough vitamin K. Another benefit of this vitamin is that it slows aging in the brain.

Capers

Frequently found in Mediterranean dishes, capers are immature flower buds that have been pickled. They have long been used throughout the world in ancient medicine, and now studies have proven that they are indeed great for health.

Liver disease is a prominent condition that can affect people due to either excessive alcohol consumption or excess fat gained in the liver. Even if a person is thin, they may develop non-alcoholic liver disease. If their liver is simply predisposed to gaining weight despite being an overall healthy weight. Thankfully, one study found that when a person consumes forty to fifty grams of capers daily, they can reduce the severity of their liver disease.

Extra Virgin Olive Oil

Olive oil is a notoriously heart-healthy source of fat, as it is largely made up of an incredible monounsaturated, known as oleic acid. This is the same type of fats that avocados are known for. This type of fat has been extensively studied and found to treat everything from skin conditions to cancer. Not only are these all great reasons to make the switch to extra virgin olive oil, but it is also resistant to heat, meaning it is useful in cooking.

Parsley

People usually only think of herbs as a source of flavor and not one for vitamins and minerals. But, parsley will surprise you! It is high in vitamins C, K, A, folate, and potassium.
Vitamin K plays an important role in bone health.

You can't just depend on calcium to take care of your bones, as it takes many vitamins and minerals to keep your skeleton strong. The great news is that a single half cup of parsley contains a shocking five-hundred and forty-seven percent of your daily intake requirements.

Celery

Celery might be incredibly low in calories, with only ten calories per stalk, but this crispy and fresh vegetables have many benefits aside from reducing your caloric intake. For instance, celery has approximately twenty-five different anti-inflammatory compounds in it, allowing it to greatly reduce inflammation all throughout the body, especially if enjoyed regularly.

Matcha Green Tea

Matcha can greatly help liver health, allowing you to reduce the risk of disease and better remove toxins from your bloodstream. Not only is this helpful for people with liver disease, but it is also good news for the elderly and those with diabetes.

After twelve weeks of regular consumption, people experienced a significant decrease in the liver enzyme levels that indicate liver damage in a scientific study. Matcha, much like coffee, can also improve brain function such as memory, reaction time, attention, and alertness.

Bird's Eye Chilies

A single tablespoon of chilies contains your daily requirements of vitamin C. This is not only great for your overall health and immune system, but it can also improve your hair and skin through its ability to strengthen collagen.

Radicchio

Also known as red chicory and red endive, radicchio (like all other sirtfoods) has many health benefits to boast of. This is in part due to the concentration of sirtuins in the food, but also due to other high levels of nutrients. You can get plenty of vitamin K and antioxidants, along with a decent amount of vitamin E, potassium, folate, vitamin C, copper, and fiber.

The nutrients in radicchio have been found to help moderate blood pressure and reduce the risk of heart disease. It can also help reduce the macular degeneration that worsens eyesight and leads to cataracts.

This gorgeous vegetable can be used in salads, roasted, sautéed, or grilled. Radicchio goes great with a large number of dishes and is a tasty side dish.

Turmeric

Turmeric contains a powerful antioxidant, curcumin, that can fight and neutralize free radicals to protect your cells. But it doesn't stop there. Unlike most sources of antioxidants, curcumin goes a step further by increasing the body's production of antioxidant enzymes. This means that you can fight free radicals on multiple fronts for better results.

Walnuts

Walnuts promote healthy gut health, therefore benefiting your overall health as it has been found that your gut health determines a great deal of your well being. Studies have found that a single serving of walnuts daily can increase beneficial gut bacteria.

Blueberries

This little berry is low in calories but high in health benefits, such as its effects on the heart and the brain: two of the most vital organs.

To help your heart, regular blueberry consumption can decrease LDL cholesterol. A single serving daily over a period of eight weeks was found to decrease LDL cholesterol by a shocking twenty-seven percent in one study.

It can also reduce blood pressure by four to six percent over the same period of time. When combined, both of these effects greatly reduce a person's risk of heart disease.

Onion

Onions are another one of many sirtfoods that has a long history of being used in ancient medicine due to its profound health benefits. They have been used to treat a number of maladies such as heart disease, headaches, lung disorders, and mouth sores. Onions have been found to decrease blood sugar.

Strawberries

You can find many vitamins and minerals within strawberries, such as vitamins K and C, potassium, folate, magnesium, and manganese. These, combined with the polyphenols and other plant-based compounds, allow strawberries to boast a range of benefits.

Red Wine

Red wine promotes heart health, but it can benefit other aspects of your well being, as well. For instance, it can increase bone health, increase mental sharpness and response, and boost your gut health.

Black Currant

The high number of nutrients found in black currants can clean out your arteries to prevent life-threatening plaque buildup, lower blood pressure, decrease platelet clumping, and protect the heart's cells against damage.

Cherries

Cherries are rich and full of antioxidants, sirtuins, vitamins, and minerals, all of which give them an abundance of health benefits. One such benefit is their ability to promote your workout recovery.

Wheat Bran

Much like wheat germ, wheat bran is packed with nutrients and fiber. In fact, wheat bran is superior to the wheat germ in this sense, as it is lower in calories while containing three times the fiber.

It also contains essential B vitamins and manganese. Just adding a couple of tablespoons to your food a day, such as over some soy yogurt or in a smoothie, you can greatly benefit your health.

Wheat bran acts as a prebiotic, supporting your gut health. Studies have found that prebiotics such as this can relieve gastrointestinal disorders such as constipation, bloating and discomfort, hemorrhoids, and digestive tract infections known as diverticulitis. By increasing healthy gut bacteria, you can also boost your immune system.

Cranberries

Cranberries also prevent infection from bacteria that causes stomach inflammation, ulcers, and cancer. By consuming cranberry juice daily, you can significantly decrease your risk of stomach cancer, among other digestive and urinary tract infections and disorders.

Peanuts

Peanuts are not actually a nut and are referred to as an oilseed due to their large contents of fat. That is primarily made of monounsaturated and polyunsaturated fats in the form of oleic and linoleic acid.

This is good news, as oleic acid is the same type of heart-healthy fat that olives and avocados are famous for. The result is that just as these two other foods can help decrease cholesterol, manage blood pressure, reduce blood triglyceride levels, and improve overall heart health, so too can peanuts.

Dark Plums

Plums and prunes have long been known to have a wealth of health benefits, but frequently people only consider them for digestive health and to reduce constipation. The truth is that they contain many compounds that greatly reduces a person's likelihood of developing a number of chronic illnesses, and they can also help manage said conditions.

Cinnamon

One of the many powerful effects the cinnamon has is to reduce inflammation. This, in turn, reduces pain and the risk of developing a number of common diseases. Another powerful effect it has is in how it relates to insulin.

Many people develop a resistance to insulin, especially if they are at a heavier weight. This insulin resistance is a trademark symptom of type II diabetes. But, cinnamon can reduce this insulin resistance, allowing the hormone to do what it was meant to do.

This naturally reduces a person's risk of developing diabetes, as well as reducing weight retention.

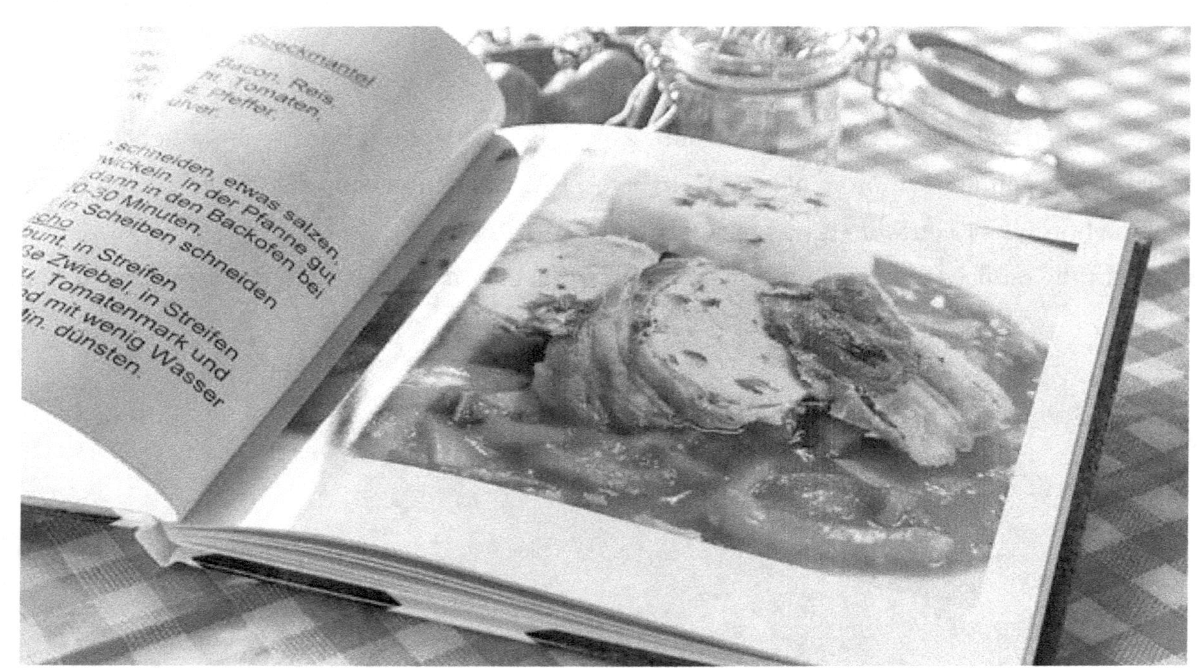

Measurement

CUP	ONCES	MILLILITERS	TABLESPOONS
8 cup	64 oz	1895 ml	128
6 cup	48 oz	1420 ml	96
5 cup	40 oz	1180 ml	80
4 cup	32 oz	960 ml	64
2 cup	16 oz	480 ml	32
1 cup	8 oz	240 ml	16
3/4 cup	6 oz	177 ml	12
2/3 cup	5 oz	158 ml	11
1/2 cup	4 oz	118 ml	8
3/8 cup	3 oz	90 ml	6
1/3 cup	2.5 oz	79 ml	5.5
1/4 cup	2 oz	59 ml	4
1/8 cup	1 oz	30 ml	3
1/16 cup	1/2 oz	15 ml	1

Temperature

FAHRENHEIT	CELSIUS
100 °F	37 °C
150 °F	65 °C
200 °F	93 °C
250 °F	121 °C
300 °F	150 °C
325 °F	160 °C
350 °F	180 °C
375 °F	190 °C
400 °F	200 °C
425 °F	270 °C
450 °F	230 °C
500 °F	260 °C
525 °F	274 °C
550 °F	288 °C

Weight

IMPERIAL	METRIC
1/2 oz	15 g
1 oz	29 g
2 oz	57 g
3 oz	85 g
4 oz	113 g
5 oz	141 g
6 oz	170 g
8 oz	227 g
10 oz	283 g
12 oz	340 g
13 oz	369 g
14 oz	397 g
15 oz	425 g
1 lb	453 g

Symbols Legend

 **Preparation Time**

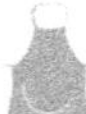 **Cooking Time**

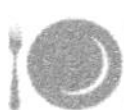 **Servings**

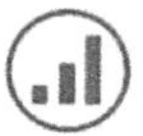 **Nutrition Facts**

Chapter 7

Breakfast

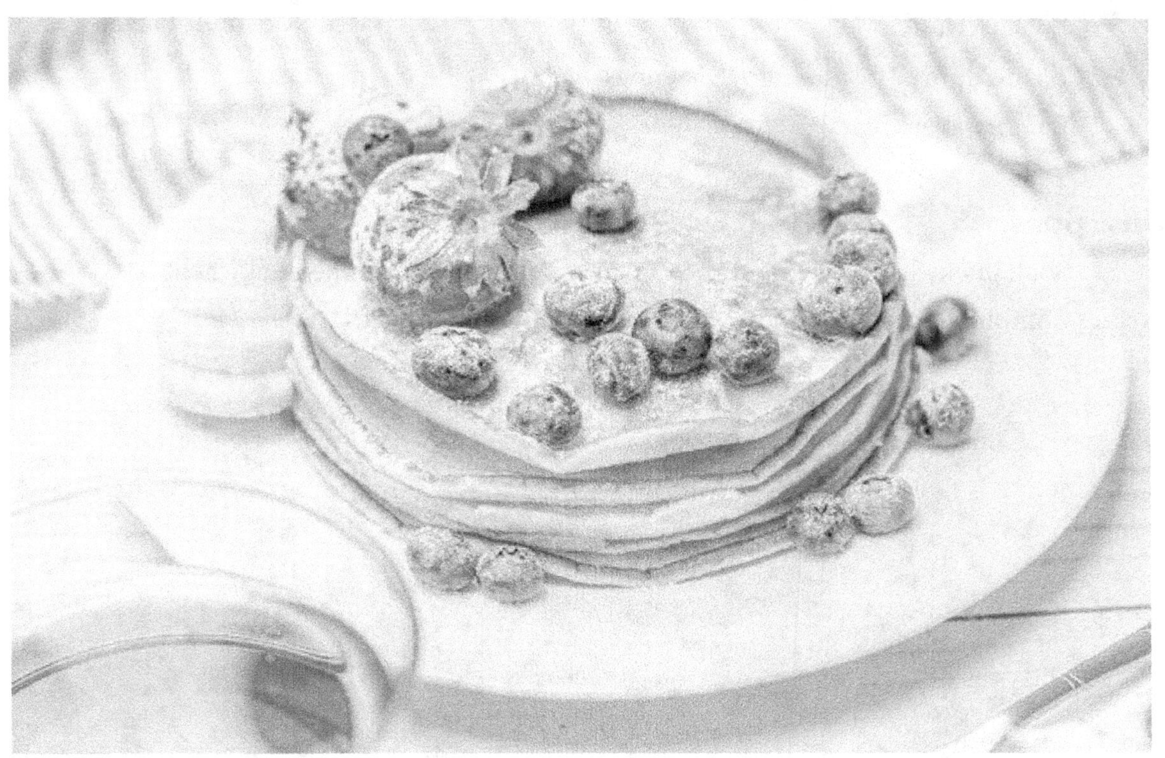

Ingredients:

- 1/2 cup Buckwheat
- 1/2 cup milk, 2%
- 1/2 cup water
- 1 medium (7" to 7-7/8" long) Banana, fresh
- 1 tbsp Peanut Butter, smooth style, with salt
- 1 tbsp Coconut Flakes

Directions:

1. Soak buckwheat overnight the morning drain and rinse the buckwheat
2. Combine ingredient microwave for 1- 1.5 minutes

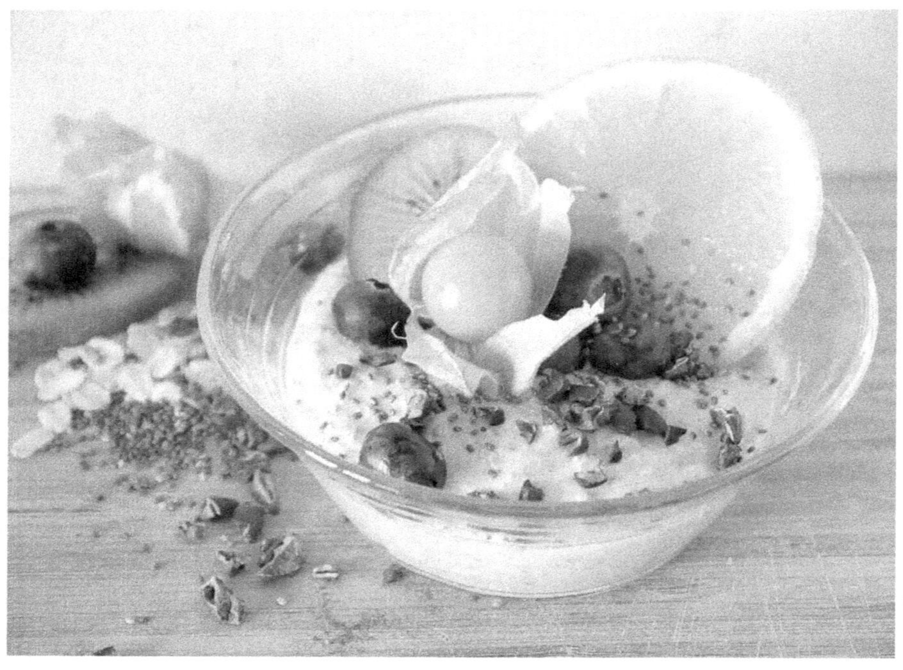

 **5 mins** 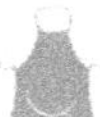 **5 mins** 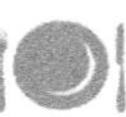 1 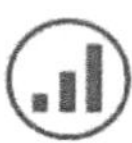

Calories: 190 - Fat: 2.1g - Fiber: 4g

Carbs: 40g - Protein: 4.1g

Ingredients:

- 1 tsp ($^{1/2}$ fl oz – 15 ml) olive oil
- 1 shallot, peeled and finely chopped
- 2 large eggs, at room temperature
- Handful (1 oz – 20 g) rocket leaves
- Small handful (1/2 oz – 10 g) parsley, finely chopped
- Salt and freshly ground black pepper

Directions:

1. In a wide frying pan: heat the oil on medium-low heat and gently fry the shallot for 5 minutes. Turn the heat up a little bit and cook for another 2 minutes.

2. In a bowl or cup, whisk the eggs together well with a fork. Distribute the shallot evenly around the pan before pouring m the eggs. Tip the pan slightly to each side so that the egg is evenly distributed. Cook for a minute or so before lifting the sides of the omelet and letting any runny egg slip into the base of the pan. Immediately sprinkle over the rocket leaves and parsley and season generously with salt and pepper.

3. When cooked, the top of the omelet will still be soft but not runny, and the base will be just starting to brown. Tip onto a plate and enjoy straight away.

 **5 mins** 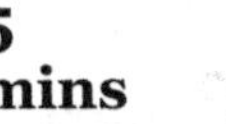 **5/10mins** 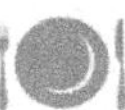 1 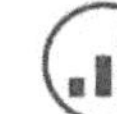 Calories: 220 - Fat: 3.4g - Fiber: 4.4g
Carbs: 48g - Protein: 6g

Ingredients:

- 1/3 oz (20 g) buckwheat flakes
- 1/3 oz (10 g) buckwheat puffs
- 1/2 oz (15 g) coconut flakes or dried coconut
- 1 ½ oz (40 g) Medjool dates, pitted and chopped
- 1/2 oz (15 g) walnuts, chopped
- 1/3 oz (10 g) cocoa nibs
- 3 ½ oz (100 g) strawberries, hulled and chopped
- 3 ½ oz (100 g) plain Greek yogurt (or vegan alternative, such as soy or coconut yogurt)

Directions:

1. Mix all of the ingredients together (leave out the strawberries and yogurt if not serving right away).

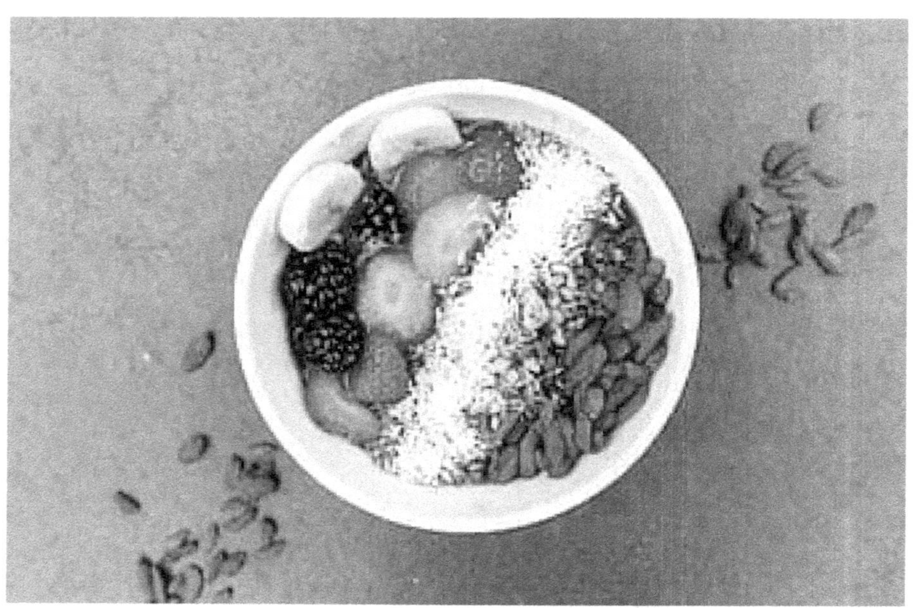

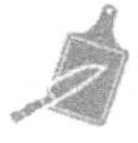 **5 mins** 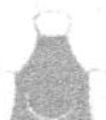 **0 mins**  1 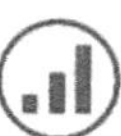 Calories: 176 - Fat: 2.1g - Fiber: 3.2g
Carbs: 3.4g - Protein: 5g

Ingredients:

- Optional* Add a seed mixture as a topper and some Rooster Sauce for flavor
- ½ oz (5 g) of finely chopped parsley
- A handful of thinly sliced button mushrooms
- ½ thinly sliced bird's eye chili
- 1 tsp (½ fl oz – 15 ml) extra virgin olive oil
- 1 oz (20 g) of kale, roughly chopped
- 1 tsp of mild curry powder
- 1 tsp of ground turmeric
- 2 eggs

Directions:

1. Mix together the curry powder, turmeric, and a small splash of water to form a light paste. Add the kale to a steamer basket and steam in boiling water for 2– 3 minutes.
2. Heat the oil over medium heat in a frying pan and fry mushrooms and chili for 2 to 3 minutes until soft and starting to brown.

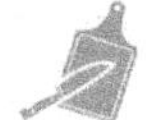 5 mins 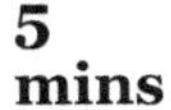 5 mins 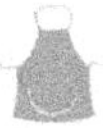 1 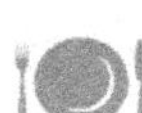 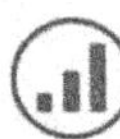

Calories: 198 - Fat: 2.4g - Fiber: 3.2g
Carbs: 39g - Protein: 5.1g

Ingredients:

- Salt, pepper
- 1 tablespoon of hemp seed
- 1 tablespoon of pumpkin seed
- 2 tablespoon of nutritional yeast
- 1 tablespoon of sun-dried tomato-walnut pesto
- 1 teaspoon of tahini
- 1 scallion
- 1 cup of sliced cherry tomatoes
- 1 cup of chopped kale
- 1 teaspoon of dried basil
- 1 ½ teaspoons of dried oregano
- 1 ½ -2 cups of veggie stock (or water)
- ½ cup of couscous
- ½ cup of oats

Directions:

1. In a small cooking pot, add oats, oregano, vegetable stock, basil, couscous, pepper, and salt and cook for about 5 minutes on medium heat frequently stirring until porridge is creamy and soft.
2. Add chopped kale but reserve a bit for garnish, tomatoes, and sliced scallion.
3. Cook for an additional 1 minute, stir in pesto, tahini, and nutritional yeast.
4. Top with the reserved kale, pumpkin and hemp seeds plus cherry tomatoes, Enjoy!

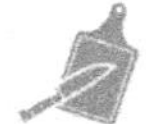 **5 mins**

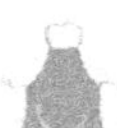 **5/10 mins**

 1

Calories: 188 - Fat: 2.8g - Fiber: 3.6g
Carbs: 34.9g - Protein: 5g

Ingredients:

- 1 cup plain Greek yogurt
- 1 garlic clove, minced
- 1 to 2 tablespoons lemon juice (from 1 lemon), to taste
- ¼ teaspoon ground turmeric
- 10 fresh mint leaves, minced
- 2 teaspoons lemon zest (from 1 lemon)

For the Pancakes

- 2 teaspoons ground turmeric
- 1½ teaspoons ground cumin
- 1 teaspoon salt
- 1 teaspoon ground coriander
- ½ teaspoon garlic powder
- ½ teaspoon freshly ground black pepper 1 head broccoli, cut into florets
- 3 large eggs, lightly beaten
- 2 tablespoons (1 fl oz – 30 ml) plain unsweetened almond milk 1 cup almond flour
- 4 teaspoons (2 fl oz – 60 ml) coconut oil

Directions:

1. Make the yogurt sauce. Combine the yogurt, garlic, lemon juice, turmeric, mint, and zest in a bowl. Taste and season with more lemon juice, if needed. Set aside or refrigerate until ready to serve.

2. Make the pancakes. In a small bowl, combine the turmeric, cumin, salt, coriander, garlic, and pepper. Place the broccoli in a food processor and pulse until the florets are broken up into small pieces. Transfer the broccoli to a large bowl and add the eggs, almond milk, and almond flour. Stir in the spice mix and combine well. Heat 1 teaspoon of the coconut oil in a nonstick pan over medium-low heat.

3. Pour ¼ cup batter into the skillet. Cook the pancake until small bubbles begin to appear on the surface, and the bottom is golden brown, 2 to 3 minutes. Flip over and cook the pancake for 2 to 3 minutes more.

4. To keep warm, transfer the cooked pancakes to an oven-safe dish and place it in a 200°F oven. Continue making the remaining 3 pancakes, using the remaining oil and batter.

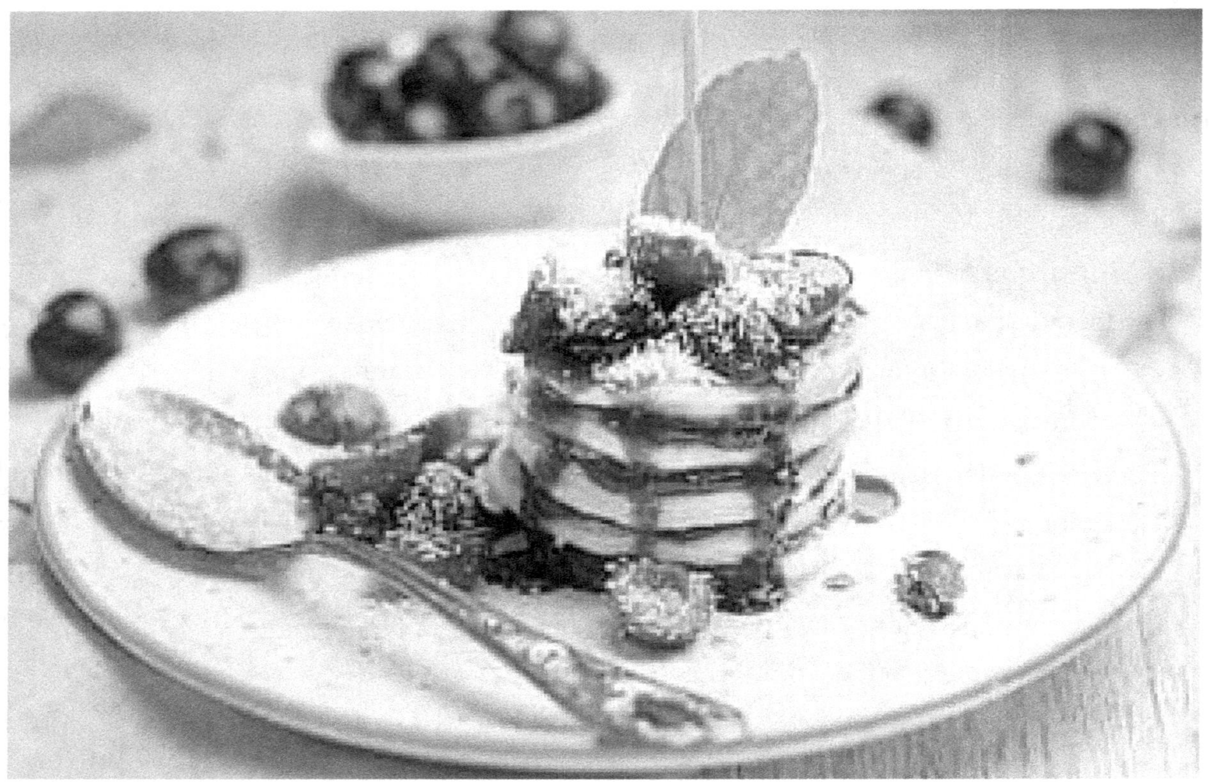

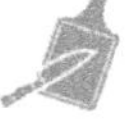 **5 mins**   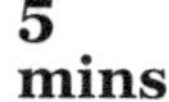 **10 mins**   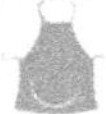 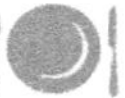 1   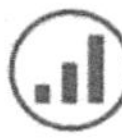   Calories: 290 - Fat: 4.35g - Fiber: 3.7g
Carbs: 45.8g - Protein: 4.9g

Ingredients:

- Language muffin - I enjoy Ezekiel 7 grain
- egg-whites - 6 tbsp or two large egg whites
- turkey bacon or bacon sausage
- sharp cheddar cheese or gouda
- green berry
- Toppings: lettuce, and hot sauce, hummus, flaxseeds, etc.

Directions:

1. At a microwavable safe container, then spray entirely to stop the egg from adhering, then pour egg whites into the dish.
2. Lay turkey bacon or bacon sausage paper towel and then cook.
3. Subsequently, toast your muffin, if preferred.
4. Then put the egg dish in the microwave for 30 minutes. Afterward, with a spoon or fork, then immediately flip egg within the dish and cook for another 30 minutes.
5. While dish remains hot sprinkle some cheese while preparing sausage.
6. The secret is to get a paste of some kind between each coating to put up the sandwich together, i.e., a very small little bit of hummus or even cheese.

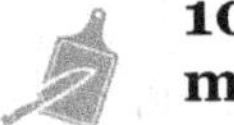 **10 mins** 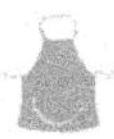 **60 mins** 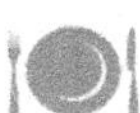 4

Calories: 214 - Fat: 3.6g - Fiber: 5.5g
Carbs: 40g - Protein: 5g

Ingredients:

- 2 Medium eggs
- 3½ oz (100 g) Smoked salmon, cut.
- Capers 1/2 tsp,
- ½ oz (5/10 g) Rocket, chopped,
- 1 tsp Parsley, chopped,
- 1 tsp (½ fl oz – 15 ml) of olive oil extra virgin,

Directions:

1. Crack the eggs in a bowl and whisk fine. Attach the salmon, capers, parsley, and rocket.
2. In a non-stick frying pan, heat the olive oil until hot but not smoking.
3. Add the egg mixture and transfer the dough around the pan, using a spatula or fish slice until it is even. Reduce heat, and cook through the omelets.
4. Slide the spatula around the edges and roll the omelets up or fold in half to serve.

 **10 mins**  **60 mins** 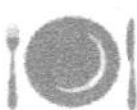 **4** 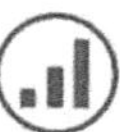

Calories: 315 - Fat: 6g - Fiber: 7g
Carbs: 70g - Protein: 7g

Ingredients:

- 2¹ᐟ² oz (75 g) of porridge oats,
- 1 tsp of baking powder,
- 2 tbsp of caster sugar,
- Two apples, peeled, cored and cut into small pieces,
- 10 fl oz (300 ml) of semi-skimmed milk,
- 2 tsp (1 fl oz – 30 ml) of light olive oil,
- For the compote:
- 4¹ᐟ² oz (120 g) of blackcurrant,
- Washed and removed stalks, 2 tbsp.
- 3 Tbsp caster sugar.

Directions:

1. Render the compote, first. In a small casserole, put the blackcurrants, sugar, and water. Bring to a cooker and boil for 10-15 minutes.

2. In a large bowl, add the oats, flour, baking powder, caster sugar, and salt and combine well. Stir in the apple and whisk a little at a time in the milk until you have a smooth blend. Whisk the egg whites to stiff peaks, then fold into the batter for the pancake.

3. Bring the mixture over to a tub. Heat 1/2 tsp of oil over medium-high heat in a non-stick frying pan and pour approximately one-quarter of the mixture.

4. Cook until golden brown, on both sides. Cut for four pancakes and repeat to make.

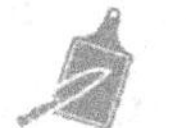 **10 mins** 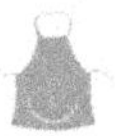 **20 mins**   1  Calories: 317 - Fat: 10g - Fiber: 8,4g
Carbs: 80g - Protein: 4g

Ingredients:

- 1 teaspoon (¹/₃ fl oz – 10 ml) additional virgin olive oil
- 1/3 oz (20 g) red onion, finely slashed
- ½ Thai chili, finely cleaved
- 3 medium eggs
- ¼ cup (1½ fl oz – 50 ml) milk
- 1 teaspoon ground turmeric
- 1/6 oz (5 g) parsley, finely slashed

Directions:

1. Warmth the oil in a griddle and fry the red onion and bean stew until delicate, however not sautéed. Whisk together the eggs, milk, turmeric, and parsley.
2. Add to the hot skillet and keep cooking over low to medium warmth, continually moving the egg blend around the dish to scramble it and prevent it from staying/consuming.
3. At the point when you have accomplished your ideal consistency, serve.

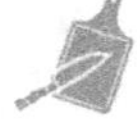 **5 mins** 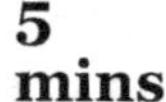 **10 mins** 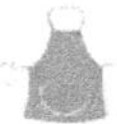 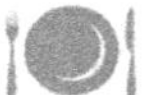 1 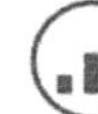

Calories: 190 - Fat: 2,6g - Fiber: 3,2g
Carbs: 29,9g - Protein: 3,1g

Ingredients:

- 1¹ᐟ² oz (50 g) cheddar cheese, grated
- 2¹ᐟ² oz (75 g) kalamata olives pitted and halved
- 8 cherry tomatoes, halved
- 4 large eggs
- 1 tbsp fresh parsley, chopped
- 1 tbsp fresh basil, chopped
- 1 tbsp (½ fl oz – 15 ml) olive oil

Directions:

1. Whisk eggs together in a large mixing bowl. Toss in the parsley, basil, olives, tomatoes, and cheese, stirring thoroughly.
2. In a small skillet, heat the olive oil over high heat. Pour in the frittata mixture and cook for 5-10 minutes, or set.
3. Remove the skillet from the hob and place under the grill for 5 minutes, or until firm and set.
4. Divide into portions and serve immediately.

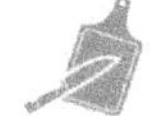 **5 mins** 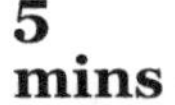 **10 mins** 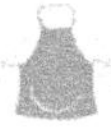 **1** 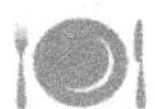 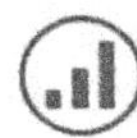

Calories: 220 - Fat: 3,2g - Fiber: 2,9g
Carbs: 45,3g - Protein: 3,8g

Ingredients:

- ½ cup quinoa
- 1 cup (8 fl oz- 240 ml) milk
- 2-3 tbsp honey, optional
- 1 tsp cinnamon
- ½ tsp vanilla
- 1 tsp ground flaxseed
- 2 tbsp walnuts or almonds, chopped
- 2 tbsp dried cranberries

Directions:

1. Rinse quinoa and drain.
2. Combine milk, quinoa, and flaxseed into a saucepan.
3. Bring to a boil, add in cinnamon and vanilla and simmer for about 15 minutes.
4. When done, place a portion of the quinoa into a bowl, drizzle with honey, and top with cranberries and crushed walnuts.

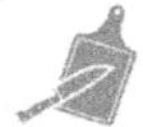 **5 mins** 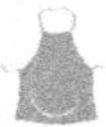 **15/20 mins** 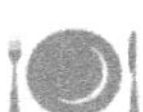 **1** 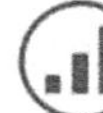

Calories: 289 - Fat: 4,5g - Fiber: 3,9g
Carbs: 59,8g - Protein: 4,9g

Ingredients:

- 1 cup of strawberries, chopped
- 1 cup of oats
- ½ cup (4 fl oz – 120 ml) of milk
- ½ cup (4 fl oz – 120 ml) of green tea
- ¼ cup walnuts, crushed (optional)

Directions:

1. Cooking with green tea is a great way to add the health benefits of this incredible beverage to meals without any added effort. Green tea oatmeal will have slightly more depth to the flavor, but little other noticeable characteristics, beyond the benefits to your health.
2. Add green tea, oats, walnuts, and milk to a pot.
3. Stir over low heat until the oatmeal becomes thick (according to your package) and then remove the saucepan from heat.
4. Divide the oatmeal between 4 bowls and top with strawberries.

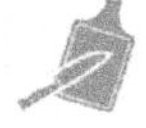 **5 mins** 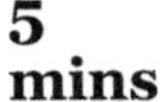 **15 mins**  1 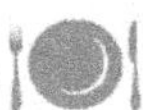 

Calories: 200 - Fat: 3,5g - Fiber: 6g
Carbs: 35,6g - Protein: 3,7g

Ingredients:

- For the Golden Turmeric Latte:
- Turmeric powder - 1 teaspoon
- Coconut milk - 3 cups (24 fl oz – 720 ml)
- A tiny piece of fresh, peeled ginger root
- Cinnamon powder - 1 teaspoon
- Pinch of black pepper (for easy absorption)
- Raw honey or maple syrup - 1 teaspoon
- Pinch of cayenne pepper (optional)
- For the Chunky Apple Compote
- Bananas - 6
- Apples – 2 (cored and chopped roughly)
- Lemon Juice - 1 Tablespoon ($^{1/2}$ fl oz – 15 ml)
- Dates - 5 (Pitted)
- Pinch of Salt
- Cinnamon Powder - ¼ Teaspoon
- For the Blueberry Banana Pancakes
- Rolled Oats – 1 cup
- Eggs - 6
- Salt - ¼ Teaspoon
- Baking Powder - 2 Teaspoon
- Blueberries – ¼ cup

Directions:

1. For the Golden Turmeric Latte
2. Add all the ingredients for the turmeric latte into a high-speed blender. Blend until smooth.
3. Transfer the mixture into a small pan and heat over medium heat for approx four minutes until hot but not boiling.
4. For the Chunky Apple Compote
5. Add all the ingredients for the compote into the food processor, along with two tablespoons of water.
6. Pulse to get your chunky apple compote
7. For the Blueberry Banana Pancakes

8. Add the rolled oats into a high-speed blender. Pulse for a minute or until the oat flour forms. You need to ensure that your blender is very dry before adding the oats to prevent it from being soggy.

9. Add the baking powder, eggs, salt, and bananas to the blender and pulse for another two minutes until you get a smooth batter.

10. Transfer the batter to a large bowl and fold in the blueberries. Set aside to rest for ten minutes to activate the baking powder.

11. Now add a dollop of butter to your frypan on medium-high heat. Add few spoons of the blueberry pancake mix and fry until it turns golden on one side, then toss to the other side and fry to golden.

12. Spoon each batch of the mixture until you have enough pancakes. Enjoy!

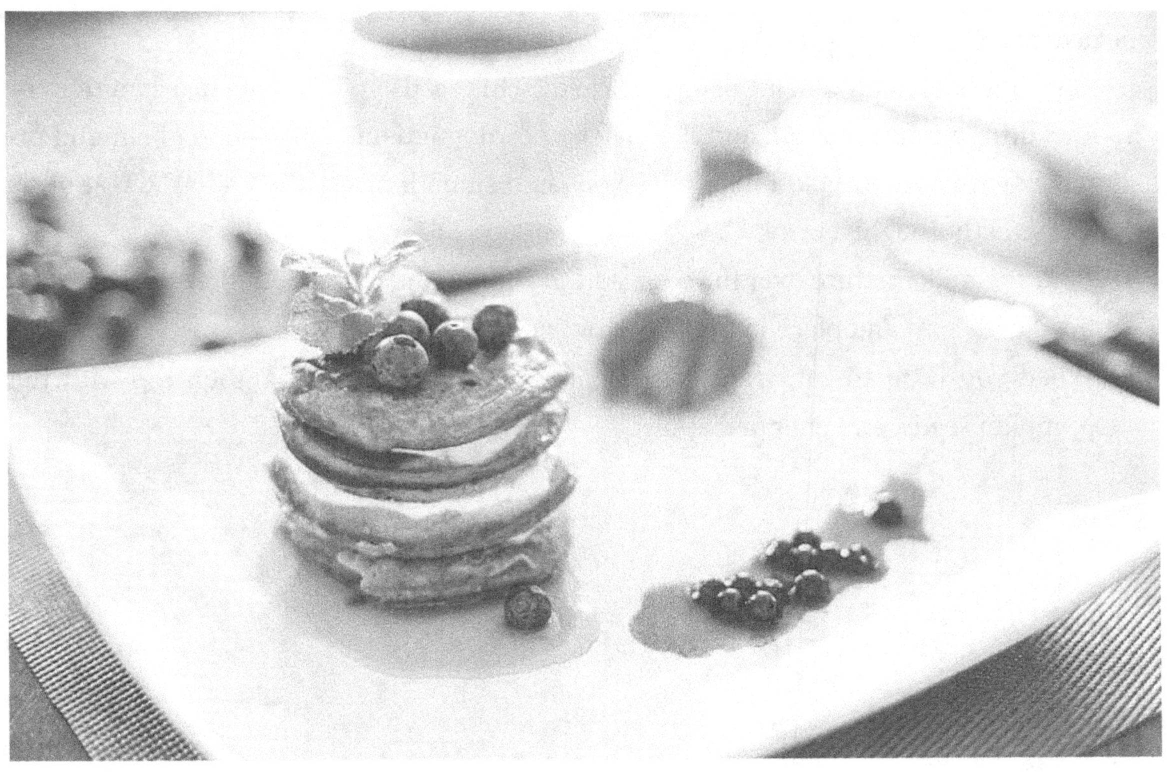

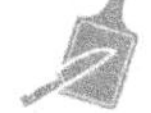 **20 mins** 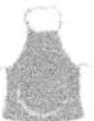 **15 mins**  1 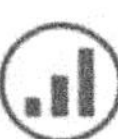 Calories: 237 - Fat: 5,8g - Fiber: 8g
Carbs: 69g - Protein: 5,7g

Ingredients:

- For the Oats
- Chia seeds - 2 teaspoon
- Rolled oats – 3 oz (85 g)
- Matcha powder - 1 teaspoon
- Honey or maple syrup - 1 teaspoon
- Ground cinnamon - 2 pinches
- Almond milk – 1 ½ cups (12 fl oz - 360 ml)
- For the Topping
- Apple – 1 (peeled, cored and chopped)
- A handful of mixed nuts
- Pumpkin seeds – 1 teaspoon

Directions:

1. Get your oats ready a night before. Place the chia seeds and the oats in a container or bowl.
2. In a different jug or bowl, add the matcha powder and one tablespoon of almond milk and whisk with a hand-held mixer until you get a smooth paste, then add the rest of the milk and mix thoroughly.
3. Pour the milk mixture over the oats, add the honey and cinnamon, then stir well. Cover the bowl with a lid and place in the fridge overnight.
4. When you want to eat, transfer the oats to two serving bowls, then top with the nuts, pumpkin seeds, and chopped apple.

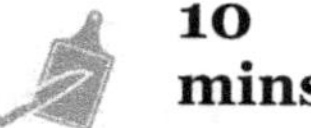 **10 mins** 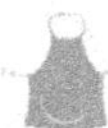 **15 mins** 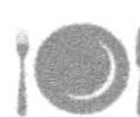 1 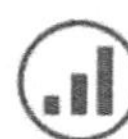 Calories: 220 - Fat: 4,5g - Fiber: 7g
Carbs: 45,8g - Protein: 8g

Chapter 8

Light Bites: Salad

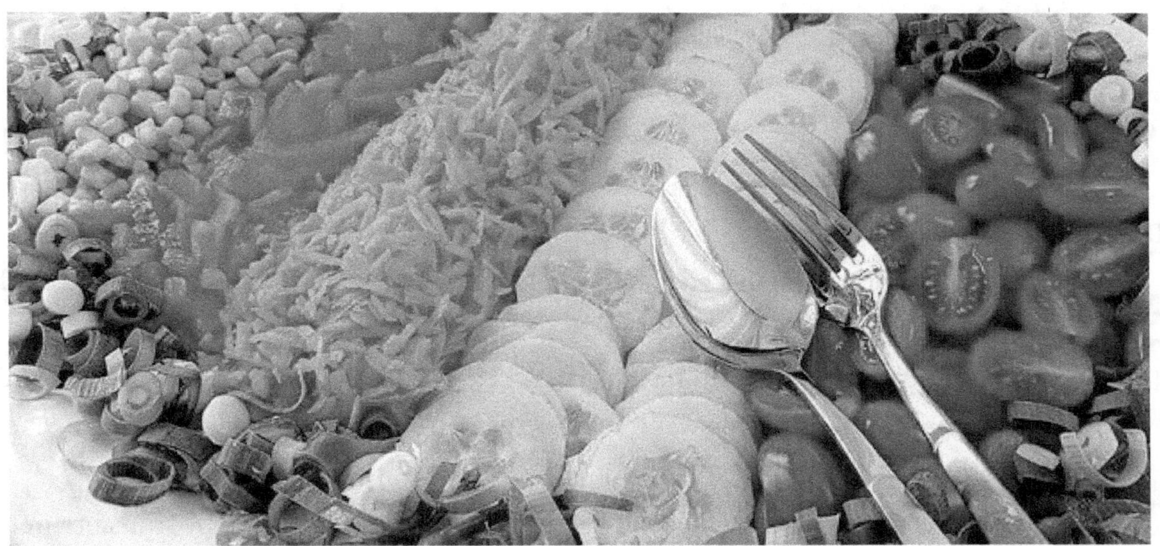

SESAME CUCUMBER SALAD

Ingredients:

- 1 lb. (450 g) Persian cucumbers
- 2 tbsp (0,3 fl oz – 10 ml) sesame oil
- 1 tbsp. sesame seeds
- 1/2 tbsp (¼ fl oz – 8 ml) lemon juice
- Kosher salt
- honey
- 1/3 cup cilantro, roughly chopped
- 1 tbsp (½ fl oz – 15 ml) low-sodium soy sauce
- 1 tsp grated peeled fresh ginger
- Chili oil, for serving

Directions:

1. Take cucumbers and halve each of them lengthwise and bash it slightly to crush, then cut each half into 4 to 6 chunks.
2. Transfer those cucumber chunks into a bowl and add 2 tsp salt. Keep it aside 10 minutes.
3. In the meantime, add it together, honey, sesame seeds, oil, ginger, soy sauce, and lemon juice together.
4. Rinse the cucumbers and shake off the water as much as possible by transferring them in a colander. Finely, add to the bowl with dressing and toss to combine, then toss with cilantro.
5. Serve drizzled with chili oil.

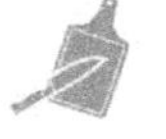 **15 mins** 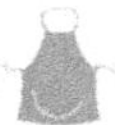 **0 mins** 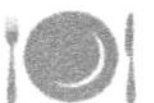 2

Calories: 180 - Fat: 2,1g - Fiber: 4,3g

Carbs: 29,9g - Protein: 3g

ROCKET SALAD WITH TUNA

Ingredients:

- 4 slices rustic bread, torn into pieces
- 4 large tomatoes
- 2 Tbsp (1 fl oz – 30 ml) olive oil
- 14 oz (400 g) tin cannellini beans drained and rinsed
- ¼ cup Kalamata olives
- 2 cups shredded rocket

- ¼ red onion, sliced finely
- 3 oz (85 g) tin tuna
- Dressing
- 2 Tbsp (1 fl oz – 30 ml) olive oil
- ½ tsp dijon mustard
- 1 Tbsp (½ fl oz – 15 ml) lemon juice

Directions:

1. Start with setting the oven at 660° F (350 °C).
2. Place the bread slices in a baking tray, put olive oil on slices, and bake for 10-15 mins.
3. To prepare the dressing mix, lemon juice, mustard, and oil in a jar.
4. Bring a bowl, add baked bread, onions, beans, tuna, tomatoes, and rocket.
5. Put the dressing over salad and enjoy.

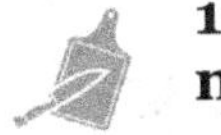 10 mins

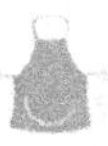 10/15 mins

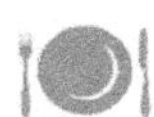 2

Calories: 195 - Fat: 2,1g - Fiber: 6g
Carbs: 40,9g - Protein: 8,5g

Ingredients:

- 3 ½ (100 g) celery including leaves, generally slashed
- 1 ½ oz (50 g) apple, generally hacked
- 1 ½ oz (50 g) pecans, generally hacked
- 1/3 oz (10 g) red onion, generally hacked
- 1/6 oz (5 g) parsley, slashed
- 1 tablespoon (½ oz – 15 ml) additional virgin olive oil
- 1 teaspoon (⅛ fl oz – 5 ml) balsamic vinegar
- juice of 1 lemon
- ¼ teaspoon Dijon mustard
- around 2 oz (50 g) arugula
- around 1 ½ oz (35 g) endive leaves

Directions:

1. Blend the celery and its leaves, apple, pecans, and onion with the parsley.
2. In a bowl, whisk the oil, vinegar, lemon juice, and mustard to make the dressing.
3. Serve the celery blend on the arugula and endive and sprinkle with the dressing.

 **5 mins** 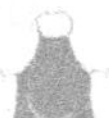 **0 mins** 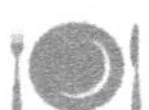 1 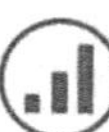 Calories: 200 - Fat: 4,9g - Fiber: 7g
Carbs: 50g - Protein: 5,3g

BUCKWHEAT PASTA SALAD

Ingredients:

- 1¹/² oz (50 g) buckwheat pasta(cooked)
- large handful of rocket
- 1/2 avocado, diced
- 8 cherry tomatoes, halved
- ¹/² oz (20 g) pine nuts
- a small handful of basil leaves
- 10 olives
- 1 tbsp (¹/² fl oz – 15 ml) extra virgin olive oil

Directions:

1. Mix all the ingredients, except for the pine nuts, gently and place on a dish or in a bowl, then spread the nuts over the edges.

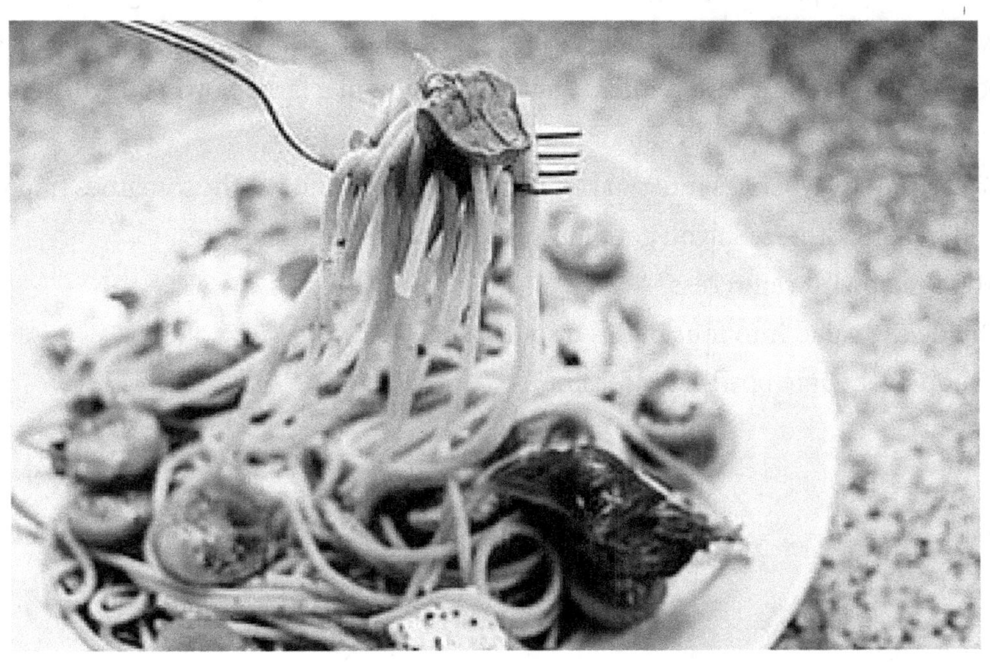

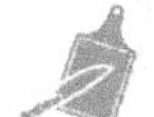 **10 mins**  **10/15 mins** 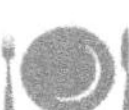 **1**  Calories: 220 - Fat: 6,7g - Fiber: 5g
Carbs: 49,7g - Protein: 7,4g

STRAWBERRY, TOMATO & WATERCRESS SALAD WITH HONEY & PINK PEPPER DRESSING

Ingredients:

- $10^{1/2}$ oz (300 g) strawberries
- 9 oz (250 g) mixed tomatoes
- $3^{1/2}$ oz (100 g) watercress, woody stalks discarded
- 1 tbsp. pink peppercorns
- ½ tbsp. honey

- 2 strawberries (about 40 g), chopped
- ½ lemon, juiced
- 3 tbsp. ($1^{1/2}$ fl oz – 45 ml) extra virgin olive oil

Directions:

1. Toast the peppercorns in a dry saucepan for 1-2 minutes until fragrant, then bash quickly with a pestle and mortar to crack the skins. Add the 2 strawberries and paste them.
2. Remove honey and lemon juice. Put the dressing in a large bowl and whisk in oil.
3. Check for seasoning, add salt or lemon juice if you prefer.
4. Break the strawberries into quarters or thin wedges and cut the tomatoes finely, slicing some and halving others, so you get plenty of different shapes.
5. Mix the bowl's watercress.
6. Divide the salad into four plates or onto a pan.
7. Spoon over some bowl-left dressing.

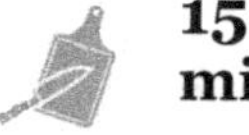 **15 mins** 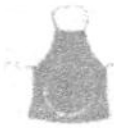 **0 mins** 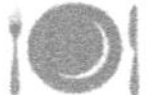 1  Calories: 278 - Fat: 8,5g - Fiber: 7,9g
Carbs: 78,9g - Protein: 5,7g

Ingredients:

- 2 pieces of skinny rice noodles
- 1/2 Tbsp (1/4 fl oz – 8 ml) sesame oil
- 2 cups Water Melon
- Head of bib lettuce
- Half of a Lot of scallions
- Half of a Lot of fresh cilantro
- 2 skinless, boneless chicken breasts
- 1/2 Tbsp Chinese five-spice
- 1 Tbsp (1/2 fl oz – 15 ml) extra virgin olive oil
- 2 Tbsp sweet skillet (I utilized a mixture of maple syrup using a dash of Tabasco)
- 1 Tbsp sesame seeds
- a couple of cashews - smashed
- Dressing - could be made daily or 2 until
- 1 Tbsp low-salt soy sauce
- 1 teaspoon (1/8 fl oz – 5 ml) sesame oil
- 1 Tbsp peanut butter
- Half of a refreshing red chili
- Half of a couple of chives
- Half of a couple of cilantro
- Inch limes - juiced
- 1 small spoonful of garlic

Directions:

1. At a bowl, then completely substituting the noodles in boiling drinking water.
2. They are going to be soon carried out in 2 minutes. On a big sheet of parchment paper, then throw the chicken with pepper, salt, and also the five-spice.
3. Twist over the newspaper, subsequently celebration and put the chicken using a rolling pin. Place into the large skillet with 1 Tbsp of olive oil, turning 3 or 4 minutes, until well charred and cooked through.
4. Drain the noodles and toss with 1 Tbsp of sesame oil onto a sizable serving dish. Place 50% the noodles into the moderate skillet, frequently stirring until crispy and nice.
5. Eliminate the Watermelon skin, then slice the flesh to inconsistent balls and then increase the platter. Reduce the lettuces and cut into small wedges and also half of a whole lot of leafy greens and scatter the dish.

6. Place another 1 / 2 the cilantro pack, the soy sauce, coriander, chives, peanut butter, and a dab of water, 1 teaspoon of sesame oil, and the lime juice then mix till smooth.

7. Set the chicken back to heat, garnish with all the sweet skillet (or my walnut syrup mixture), and toss with the sesame seeds.

8. Pour the dressing on the salad toss gently with fresh fingers until well coated, then add crispy noodles and then smashed cashews. Blend chicken pieces and add them to the salad.

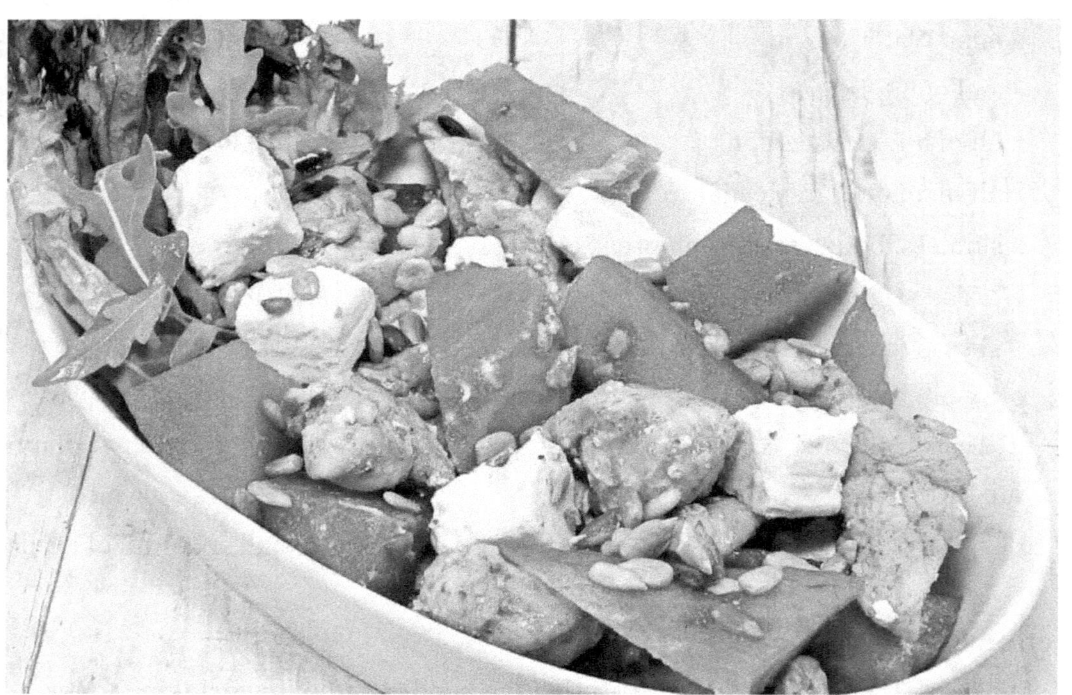

 **10 mins** 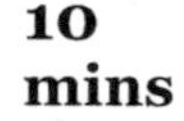 **10/15 mins** 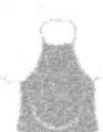 **2/4** 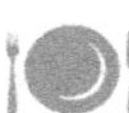  Calories: 275 - Fat: 6,4g - Fiber: 3,5g
Carbs: 76,9g - Protein: 6g

BAKED SALMON SALAD WITH CREAMY MINT DRESSING

Ingredients:

- 1 Salmon (4 ½ oz – 130 g)
- 1 ½ oz (40 g) Mixed salad leaves
- 1 ½ oz (40 g) young spinach leaves
- 2 Radishes, trimmed and thinly chopped
- 2 in (5 cm) slice (2 oz - 50 g) cucumber, cut into balls
- 2 Spring onions, trimmed and chopped
- 1 Small number (⅓ oz - 10g) parsley, roughly sliced

Dressing

- 1 Tsp low-fat mayonnaise
- 1 Tablespoons organic yogurt
- 1 Tbsp (1/2 fl oz – 15 ml) rice vinegar
- 2 Leaves mint, finely chopped
- Salt And freshly ground black pepper

Directions

1. Pre heats the oven to 400°F (350°F fan/Gas 6). Set the salmon fillet onto a baking dish and bake for 16--18 minutes until cooked. Remove from the oven and place aside.

2. The salmon is every bit as fine cold or hot in the salad. If your poultry contains skin, then just brush down the skin and eliminate the salmon out of the skin by means of a fish piece after ingestion. It will slide easily once cooked.

3. In a small bowl, add the mayonnaise, yogurt, rice vinegar, coriander leaves, and salt and salt together and leave to stand for at least 5 minutes to Permit the tastes to grow.

4. Arrange the salad lettuce and leaves onto the serving plate and top with the radishes, cucumber, spring onions, and parsley.

5. Flake the carrot on the salad and drizzle the dressing.

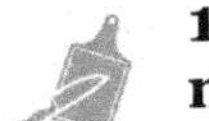 10 mins  15 mins 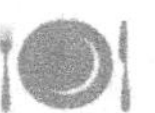 1

Calories: 289 - Fat: 4,3g - Fiber: 7,4g
Carbs: 80g - Protein: 6g

BUCKWHEAT "GARDEN" SALAD

Ingredients:

- 1 cup buckwheat groats
- 2 cups (16 fl oz – 480 ml) of water
- ½ tsp salt
- ½ chayote, finely diced
- 12 large green olives, pitted and quartered
- 1 small yellow bell pepper, diced
- 1 cup broccoli florets, chopped
- 2 oz (50g) walnut, chopped
- ¼ cup red onion, finely chopped
- ½ cup fresh dill, chopped
- 2 tbs fresh mint, chopped
- juice of 1 lime
- 2 tbsp (1 fl oz – 30 ml) white wine vinegar
- 1 tbsp (1/2 oz – 15 ml) olive oil
- ½ tsp salt
- ½ tsp black pepper

Directions:

1. In a small saucepan, bring water and salt to a boil. Add buckwheat groats, reduce heat, cover, and cook until all water has absorbed about 10 minutes.
2. Remove lid and allow to cool for at least 30 minutes. You can also cook your buckwheat groats the previous day and let them cool overnight.
3. Add all ingredients, including cooled buckwheat to a large mixing bowl.
4. Mix until well combined. Serve immediately or refrigerate for a few hours (or overnight) to allow for flavors to develop.

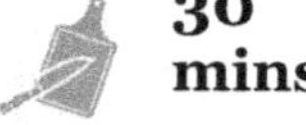 **30 mins**

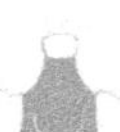 **15/20 mins**

 1

 Calories: 299 - Fat: 4,3g - Fiber: 3,2g
Carbs: 98g - Protein: 4g

SESAME CHICKEN SALAD

Ingredients:

- 1 tbsp sesame seeds
- 1 cucumber, peeled, halved lengthways, deseeded with a teaspoon and sliced
- $3^{1/2}$ oz (100 g) baby kale, roughly chopped
- 2 oz (60 g) pak choi, very finely shredded
- ½ red onion, very finely sliced
- 5 oz (150 g) cooked chicken, shredded
- 1/3 oz Large handful (20 g) parsley, chopped

For the dressing:

- 1 tbsp (1/2 fl oz – 15 ml) extra virgin olive oil
- 1 tsp (1/8 fl oz – 8 ml) sesame oil
- Juice of 1 lime
- 1 tsp clear honey
- 2 tsp (1/4 fl oz – 5 ml) soy sauce

Directions:

1. Toast the sesame seeds in a dry frying pan for 2 minutes until lightly browned and fragrant.
2. Transfer to a plate to cool. In a small bowl, mix together the olive oil, sesame oil, lime juice, honey, and soy sauce to make the dressing place the cucumber, kale, pak choi, red onion, and parsley in a large bowl and gently mix together.
3. Pour over the dressing and mix again. Distribute the salad between two plates and top with the shredded chicken.
4. Sprinkle over the sesame seeds just before serving.

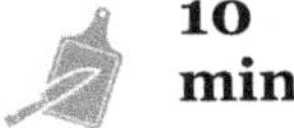 **10 mins**　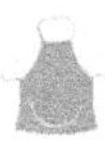 **15/20 mins**　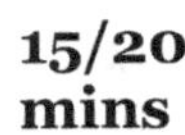 1　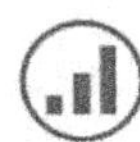 Calories: 277 - Fat: 5,4g - Fiber: 3,7g
Carbs: 76,5g - Protein: 4,9g

Chapter 9

Light Bites: Appetizers and Soups

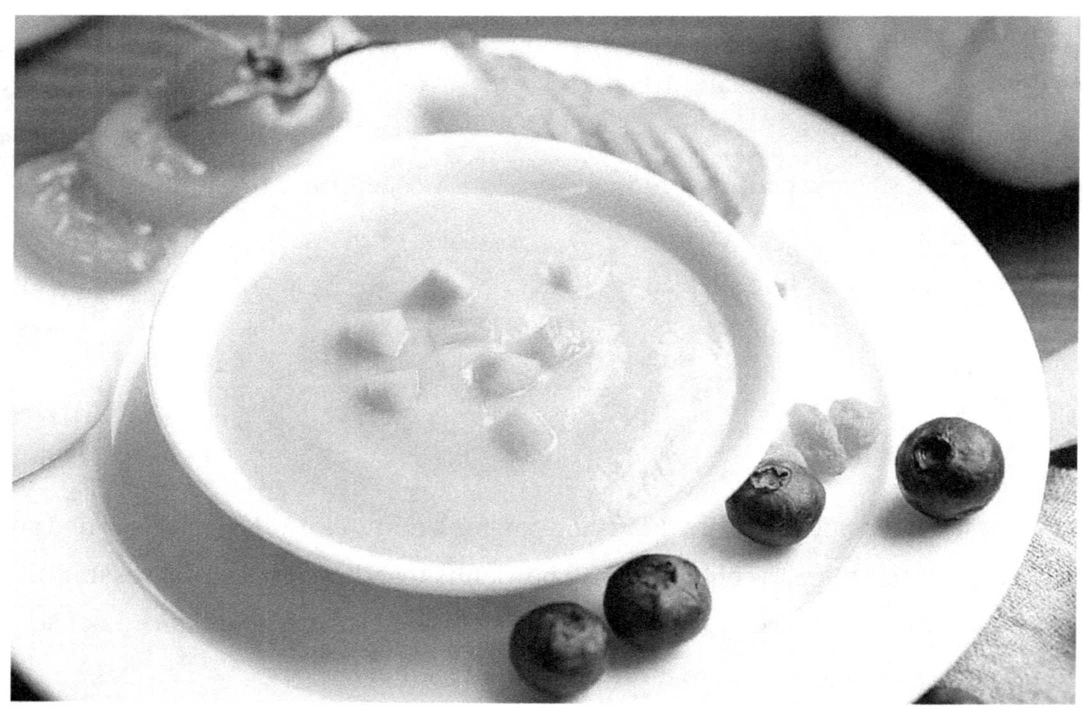

INDIAN LENTIL SOUP

Ingredients:

- 2 cups of lentils
- 1 small red onion, chopped
- 1 celery stalk, finely chopped
- 1 chopped carrot
- 2 large finely chopped kale leaves or 1 cup chopped kale
- 2 Coriander sprigs, chopped
- 3 Sprigs of chopped parsley
- ½ teaspoon salt
- 1 tomato, cut into small pieces
- ¼-1/2 hot pepper, seeded and chopped (use more or less as desired)
- 1 piece of ginger, chopped
- 1 garlic clove, chopped
- 5 cups ($5^{1/2}$ fl oz – 1200 ml) chicken or vegetable broth
- 1 teaspoon of turmeric
- 1 teaspoon (1/2 fl oz – 15 ml) extra virgin olive oil

Directions:

1. Cook the lentils according to the package and remove them from the stove about 5 minutes before finishing.
2. Fry all the vegetables in olive oil in a pan. Then add the chopped vegetables at the end. Then add the ginger, garlic, and chili and the turmeric powder.
3. Add the broth and simmer for 5 minutes. Add the lentils and salt.
4. Add the pre-cooked lentils and cook over low heat for another 25 minutes. Take it out of the stove and let it cool.
5. Cut the avocado, remove the hole and cut it, then remove the slices just before eating.
6. Cover with an avocado slice and serve immediately.

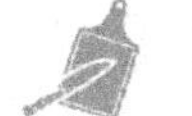 **15 mins** 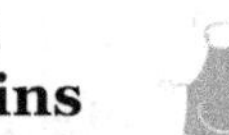 **25/30 mins** 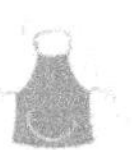 2 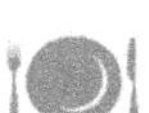 Calories: 218 - Fat: 2,9g - Fiber: 4g
Carbs: 56g - Protein: 4,8g

Ingredients:

- 1 green serrano bean stew, minced
- 1 cup cooked chickpeas
- 1/3 cup tahini
- 2 tablespoons (1 fl oz – 30ml) new lime or juice
- 4 stems of celery, cut and dig
- 1 cm pieces (around 1 cup)
- 5 tablespoons vegetable oil (ideally extra virgin olive)
- 2 cases of garlic
- 1 teaspoon salt or to taste
- 1 tablespoon minced parsley

Directions:

1. Place the celery into a heating platter. Top with 2 spoonfuls of oil.
2. Place the 2 garlic cases during a plate corner and disperse with the bean stew.
3. Bake for 45 minutes within the broiler. Bringing the chickpeas into the blender.
4. Add with any lingering oil into the blender, within the hot cooked celery and different vegetables.
5. Add the tahini, lime or lemon squeeze, salt and blend well for 3-4 minutes until smooth and sweet.
6. Remove from the blender into a bowl, mix within the staying three tablespoons of vegetable oil, and hacked parsley.

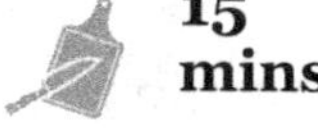 **15 mins** 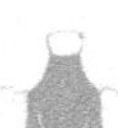 **45/50 mins**  4 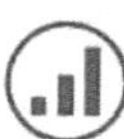 Calories: 199 - Fat: 3,8g - Fiber: 5g
Carbs: 39g - Protein: 4,8g

Ingredients:

- 3 tablespoons (1 ½ fl oz – 45ml) extra-virgin olive oil, divided
- ½ teaspoon ground pepper, divided
- 1 cup chopped spinach
- ½ cup quartered cherry tomatoes
- 1 clove garlic, minced
- ¼ teaspoon salt
- 2 tablespoons pitted and sliced Kalamata olives
- 4 portobello mushrooms
- ⅓ cup crumbled feta cheese
- 1 tablespoon chopped fresh oregano

Directions:

1. Firstly, preheat oven to 400° F (200 C°).
2. Mix 2 tablespoons oil, garlic, 1/4 teaspoon pepper, and salt in a small bowl. Using a silicone brush, coat mushrooms all over with the oil mixture.
3. Place on a large rimmed baking sheet and bake until the mushrooms are mostly soft, 8 to 10 minutes. In the meantime, combine spinach, tomatoes, feta, olives, oregano, and the remaining 1 tablespoon oil in a medium bowl.
4. Once the mushrooms have softened, remove from the oven and fill with the spinach mixture.
5. Bake until the tomatoes have wilted, about 10 minutes.

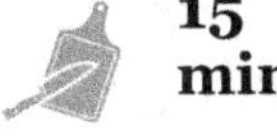 **15 mins** 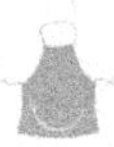 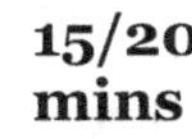 **15/20 mins** 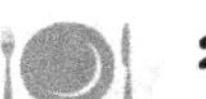 **2** 

Calories: 210 - Fat: 3,8g - Fiber: 2,8g
Carbs: 45g - Protein: 2,1g

GOLDEN CHICORY IN PROSCIUTTO WRAPS

Ingredients:

- 2 head of chicory
- 4 slices prosciutto or Serrano ham
- 2 ½ fl oz (75 ml) vegetable stock, or white wine
- 2 tablespoons butter
- 2 tablespoons Dijon mustard
- ¼ cup whipping cream
- 2 thyme sprigs
- 4 slices, about 2 oz melting cheese (cheddar is great)
- Sautéed potatoes and green salad, to serve

Directions:

1. Preheat the oven to 350° F (150 C°).
2. Cut across from the base halfway to the tip of each head of chicory.
3. Stuff the butter into the slits, then lay the slices of prosciutto or Serrano ham in pairs on the work surface, overlapping them slightly.
4. Paint the ham with the mustard and lay the chicory on top. Roll each chicory head away from you, wrapping it snugly in the ham.
5. Lay the wrapped chicory in a small ovenproof dish or pan, pour over the vegetable stock or white wine on top with the thyme sprigs. Cover the dish with a loose tent of foil and bake for 30-40 minutes until the chicory is softened.
6. Uncover the dish, lay the cheese slices over the chicory and bake, still uncovered, for a further 6-8 minutes, until the cheese is melting and golden.
7. The chicory is now ready to serve. For an extra touch, remove the chicory, place the pan on medium heat and boil the juices with the cream for 4-5 minutes until rich and syrupy.
8. Pour the sauce over the chicory. Serve with sautéed potatoes and salad.

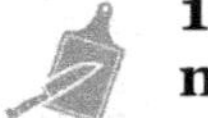 **10 mins**

 **30/40 mins**

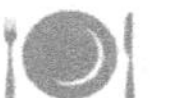 1

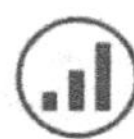 Calories: 187 - Fat: 2,8g - Fiber: 4g
Carbs: 31,5g - Protein: 3g

SHRIMP & ARUGULA SOUP

Ingredients:

- 10 medium-sized shrimp or 5 large prawns, cleaned, deshelled and deveined
- 1 small red onion, sliced very thinly
- 1 cup arugula
- 1 cup baby kale
- 2 large celery stalks, sliced very thinly
- 11 cloves of garlic, minced
- 5 sprigs of parsley, chopped
- 5 cups (5 ½ fl oz – 1200 ml) of chicken or fish or vegetable stock
- 1 tbsp (½ fl oz – 15 ml) extra virgin olive oil
- Dash of sea salt
- Dash of pepper

Directions:

1. Sauté the vegetables (not the kale or arugula just yet, however), in a stockpot, on low heat for about 2 minutes so that they are still tender and still crunchy, but not cooked quite yet.
2. You will need to save the cooking time for the next step. Add the salt and pepper.
3. Next, clean and chop the shrimp into bite-sized pieces that would be comfortable eating in a soup. Then, add the shrimp to the pot and sauté for 10 more minutes on medium-low heat. Make sure the shrimp is cooked thoroughly and is not translucent.
4. When the shrimp seems to be cooked through, add the stock to the pot and cook on medium for about 20 more minutes.
5. Remove from heat and cool before serving.

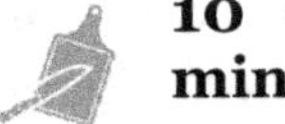 **10 mins** 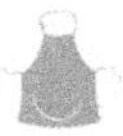 **30 mins** 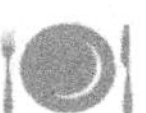 4 Calories: 210 - Fat: 5,8g - Fiber: 7g
Carbs: 67g - Protein: 7g

CHILLED GAZPACHO

Ingredients:

- 2 large, or 6 small tomatoes, chopped
- 1 avocado, pitted, sliced, and scooped out (wait to do this until instructed)
- 1 medium cucumber, chopped
- 1 small red onion, chopped
- 1 cup of arugula, chopped very finely
- ½ stalk of celery chopped very finely
- 1 clove of garlic, minced or pressed
- ½ chili or a dash of cayenne pepper
- 1 tsp (½ fl oz – 15 ml) lime juice
- Dash of sea salt
- Dash of pepper

Directions:

1. Add the ingredients to a blender or a food processor and pulse gently.
2. You do not want to blend too well, or you will make a liquid, as opposed to a soup.
3. The gazpacho should be chunky. After blending, put into the refrigerator for about 1 hour.
4. You can also let this sit overnight, just before eating, slice, and scoop out the avocado.
5. Ladle half of the gazpacho into a chilled bowl.
6. Add the slices of avocado and serve immediately.

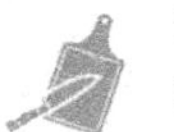 **15/20 mins** 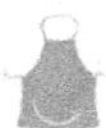 **0 mins** 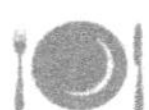 2 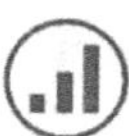 Calories: 239 - Fat: 4,3g - Fiber: 3,2g
Carbs: 54g - Protein: 4,8g

SIRT SHAKSHUKA

Ingredients:

- 1 tsp. (½ fl oz – 15 ml) extra virgin olive oil
- 1½ oz (40 g) Red onion, finely chopped
- 1 Garlic clove, finely chopped
- 1 oz (30 g) Celery, finely chopped
- 1 Bird's eye chili, finely chopped
- 1 oz (30 g) Kale, roughly chopped without stems
- 1 tsp. ground cumin
- 1 tsp. Paprika
- 1 tsp. Ground turmeric
- 14 oz (400 g) Tinned chopped tomatoes
- 1 tbsp. Chopped parsley
- 2 Medium eggs

Directions:

1. Heat a small, deep-sided pot over medium-low heat. Add oil and fry for 1–2 minutes onion, garlic, celery, chili, and spices.
2. Add tomatoes, then leave the sauce to cook for 20 minutes, stirring occasionally.
3. Add kale and cook another 5 minutes. If the sauce is too deep, easily add more water.
4. Stir in parsley when your sauce has a right, creamy consistency.
5. Create two little sauce wells and smash growing egg into them.
6. Cover with a cap or foil and lower the heat to low.
7. Leave the eggs to cook for 10–12 minutes, where the whites should be firm while the yolks are still runny.
8. Cook another 3–4 minutes if you prefer firm eggs. Serve immediately – ideally straight.

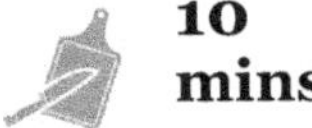 **10 mins** 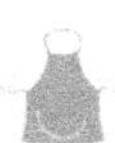 **20/25 mins**  2 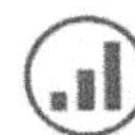 Calories: 215 - Fat: 5,7g - Fiber: 7,8g
Carbs: 76g - Protein: 5g

Ingredients:

- ¾ oz (20 g) parsley
- ¾ oz (20 g) pecans
- ¾ oz (20 g) Parmesan cheddar (or utilize a veggie lover or vegetarian elective), ground
- 1 tablespoon (½ fl oz – 15 ml) additional virgin olive oil
- juice of ½ lemon
- 3 tablespoons (1½ fl oz – 45 ml) water

- 1 little eggplant (around 5 ½ oz or 150 g), quartered
- ¾ oz (20 g) red onions, cut
- 1 teaspoon (1/8 fl oz - 5ml) red wine vinegar
- 1 oz (35 g) arugula
- 3 ½ oz (100 g) cherry tomatoes
- 1 teaspoon (1/8 fl oz - 5ml) balsamic vinegar

Directions:

1. Warmth the broiler to 400°F (200°C).
2. To make the pesto, place the parsley, pecans, Parmesan, olive oil, and a large portion of the lemon squeeze in a food processor or blender and mix until you have a smooth glue.
3. Include the water bit by bit until you have the right consistency — it ought to be sufficiently thick to adhere to the eggplant.
4. Brush the eggplant with a tad bit of the pesto, saving the rest to serve. Spot on a preparing plate and dish for 25 to 30 minutes, until the eggplant is brilliant earthy colored, delicate, and soggy.
5. In the interim, spread the red onion with the red wine vinegar and put in a safe spot—this will mollify and improve the onion. Channel the vinegar before serving.
6. Consolidate the arugula, tomatoes, and depleted onion and shower the balsamic vinegar over the plate of mixed greens.
7. Present with the hot eggplant, spooning the rest of the pesto over it.

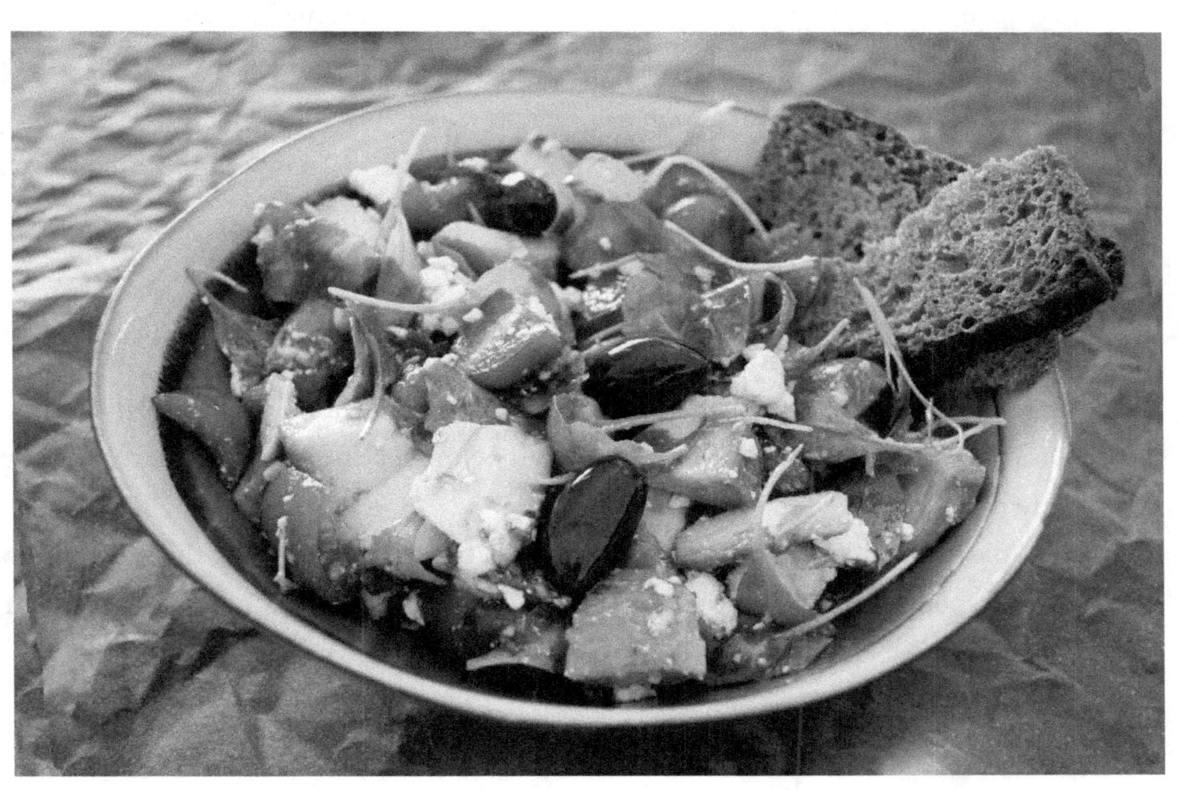

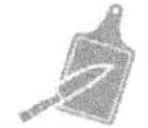 **10 mins**  **25/30 mins** 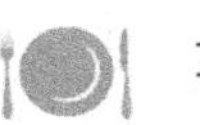 1 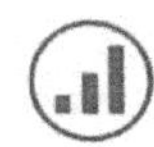 Calories: 187 - Fat: 4g - Fiber: 2,8g
Carbs: 34,8g - Protein: 4,8g

Ingredients:

- 1/3-oz (10 g) dried wakame (seaweed)
- 34 fl oz (1 liter) vegetable stock
- 7 oz (200 g) shiitake mushrooms, sliced
- 4 ½ (120 g) miso paste
- 1 x 14-ounce (400 g) block firm tofu, dig small cubes
- 2 scallions, trimmed and sliced on the diagonal
- 1 Thai chili, finely chopped (optional)

Directions:

1. Soak the wakame in warm water for 10 minutes, then drain.
2. Bring the stock to a boil, then add the mushrooms and simmer gently for 1 to 2 minutes.
3. Dissolve the miso paste during a bowl with a number of the nice and cozy stock to make sure it dissolves thoroughly.
4. Add the miso and tofu to the remaining stock, taking care not to let the soup boil as this is able to spoil the fragile miso flavor. Add the drained wakame, scallions, and chili, if using, and serve.

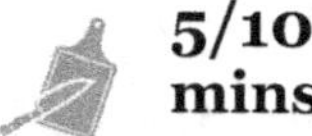 **5/10 mins**

 **20 mins**

 **2/4**

 Calories: 210 - Fat: 3g - Fiber: 4,3g
Carbs: 50g - Protein: 6g

TOFU BUCKWHEAT SOBA NOODLES CARROTS AND KALE SOUP

Ingredients:

- Salt and freshly ground black pepper
- 1 handful of chopped kale
- 2-3 finely chopped scallions
- 2 garlic cloves, minced
- 2 medium carrots, chop into small pieces
- Some chili flakes
- 3 cups (24 fl oz – 720 ml) of vegetable broth
- 2½ oz (75 g) soba (buckwheat) noodles
- 1 organic lime or lemon
- 1 tbsp (1/2 oz – 15 ml) of oil
- 7 oz (200 g) of tofu

Directions:

1. Place the tofu between two sheets of paper towel to dry off; cut into cubes. Place the tofu in a bowl and season with some chili flakes, salt, and pepper; toss to coat.
2. Heat the oil over medium heat, add the tofu and fry until all sides are golden brown.
3. Sprinkle some lime zest over. Add the vegetable broth to a pot and bring to a boil.
4. Add in the chopped carrots and cook until tender.
5. Remove carrots from the soup with a slotted spoon; Season with lots of pepper and salt. Meanwhile, cook the noodles as directed in package instructions.
6. Add the minced garlic into 2 serving bowls along with the scallions; add chopped kale, cooked carrots, tofu, noodles, and kale. Pour soup over and serve with the lime wedges.

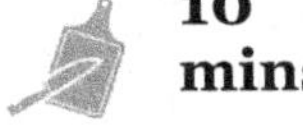 **10 mins**

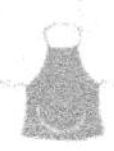 **15/20 mins**

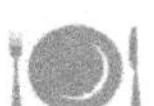 2

 Calories: 289 - Fat: 8,7g - Fiber: 7,9g
Carbs: 90g - Protein: 7,5g

Ingredients:

- 2 lemon slices
- 1 ½ fl oz (50 ml) of vegetable stock
- 1 tsp of garlic crushed
- 10 ½ oz (300 g) of king prawns raw or cooked

- 2 thinly sliced broccoli florets
- 1 stick celery
- 1 courgette
- 1 carrot, peeled
- (Optional) fresh dill

Directions:

1. Heat your oven to 350° F (180°C or 160°C fan).
2. Shave the carrot, courgette, and celery into ribbons with a veggie peeler and set aside.
3. Arrange two pieces of tin foil (large enough to hold your vegetables) add a smaller piece of greaseproof paper on top of each tin foil. Curl up edges so the filling can hold.
4. Add half of the veggies over each piece of paper; add the prawns and a slice of lemon. Mix vegetable stock with garlic and add on top the veggies.
5. Sprinkle top with dill if using. Seal the foil and transfer to the baking sheet.
6. Place the baking sheet in the oven and bake until vegetables are soft, about 10-15 minutes.
7. Remove foil and serve.

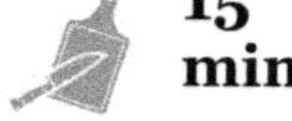 **15 mins** 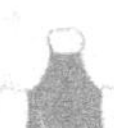 **10/15 mins** 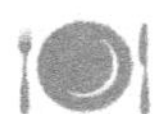 1  Calories: 235 - Fat: 4,6g - Fiber: 6,8g
Carbs: 60,5g - Protein: 7,8g

Ingredients:

- Sea salt (Himalayan, Celtic Grey, or Redmond Real Salt)
- 1 lime juice
- 1 avocado
- 8 butter lettuce leaves or romaine, these make lovely cups
- A small handful of chopped cilantro
- ¼ cup of red onion, minced
- 1 x 15-oz (425 g) can of Adzuki beans, drained and rinsed
- Red pepper flakes (optional)

Directions:

1. In a bowl, mash together the red onion and beans.
2. Add chopped cilantro, stir to combine.
3. Spoon the mash beans into lettuce cups and add diced avocado to the top with lime juice; season with red pepper flakes and salt.

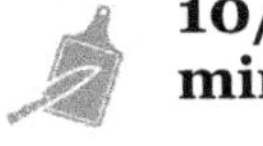 **10/15 mins** 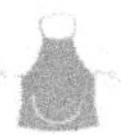 **0 mins** 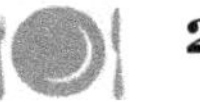 2 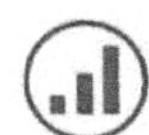 Calories: 175 - Fat: 2,1g - Fiber: 1,9g
Carbs: 28,9g - Protein: 4,5g

Chapter 10

Main Meals: Fish and Seafood

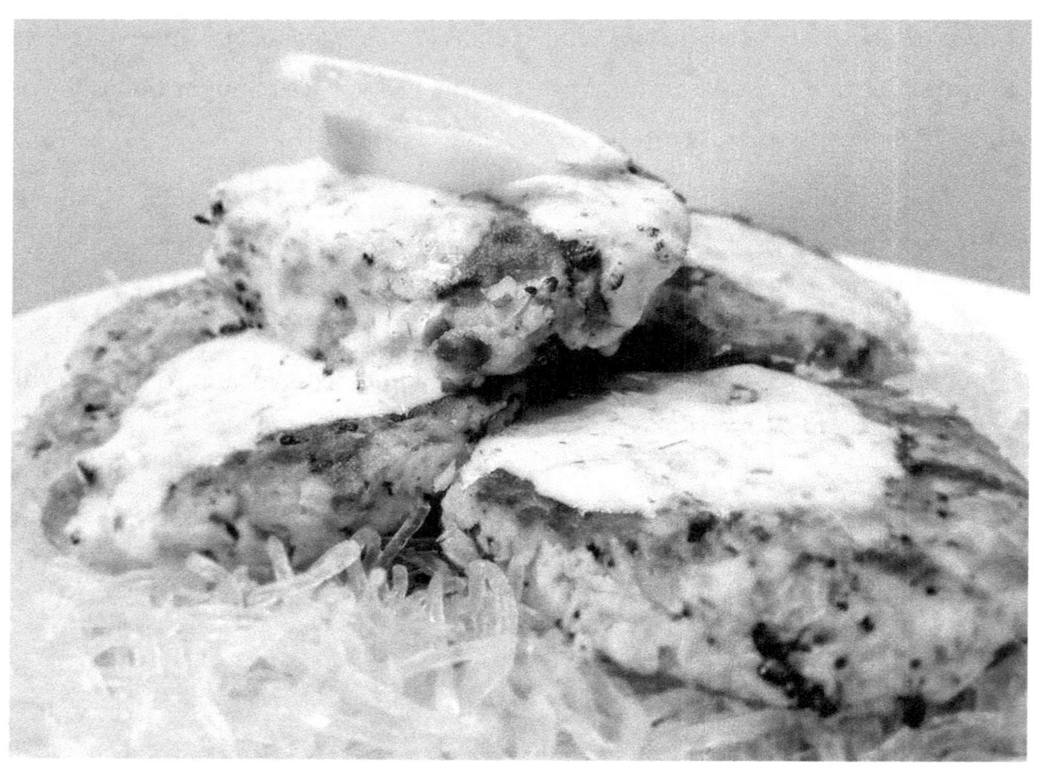

Ingredients:

- Two garlic cloves, minced
- 1 tsp. minced ginger
- 1/2 cup (4 fl oz – 120 ml) soy sauce
- 1/4 cup brown sugar
- Juice of 1 lime
- 2 tsp. (1 fl oz – 30 ml) sriracha
- Two green onions, thinly sliced

- Two green onions, thinly sliced
- 1 cup (8 fl oz – 250 ml) vegetable broth
- One large head broccoli, cut into florets
- One red bell pepper, cut into thin slices

Directions:

1. Cook ramen noodles according to package instructions.
2. In a large skillet heat vegetable oil. Add sesame oil and stir in garlic and ginger.
3. Cook until fragrant about 1 min. Add soy sauce, brown sugar, lime juice, and Sriracha. Bring mixture to a boil.
4. Add broccoli and peppers and cover the skillet cook vegetables for about 5 min.
5. Return shrimp to skillet and stir until coated in sauce.
6. Stir in cooked ramen noodles and green onions.
7. Serve with Sriracha.

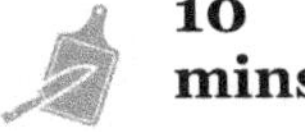 **10 mins**   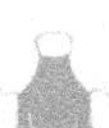 **30 mins**   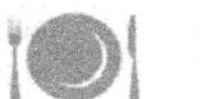 1   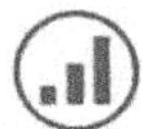 Calories: 290 - Fat: 4,3g - Fiber: 5g
Carbs: 67g - Protein: 4,8g

HONEY GLAZED SALMON

Ingredients:

- 12 oz skinless salmon (340 g)
- One tablespoon (½ fl oz – 15 ml) olive oil

- HONEY SOY MARINADE
- Two teaspoons ginger, minced
- ½ teaspoon red pepper
- One tablespoon olive oil
- ⅓ cup honey (115 g)

Directions:

1. Put salmon in a sealable bag or medium bowl. In a little bowl or cup, blend marinade ingredients.
2. Pour half marinade on the salmon.
3. Spare the other half for some additional time. Let the salmon marinate in the cooler for around 30 minutes.
4. In a medium pot, heat oil. Add salmon to the pot without marinade.
5. Cook salmon on one side for around 2-3 minutes, at that point, flip over and cook for an extra 1-2 minutes.
6. Remove salmon from the pot. Pour in excess marinade and lessen.
7. Serve the salmon with sauce. Enjoy!

 **30/40 mins** 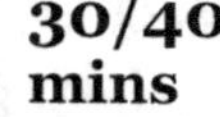 **45 mins** 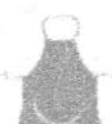 1 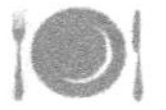 Calories: 277 - Fat: 5,6g - Fiber: 4,7g
Carbs: 67,9g - Protein: 6,5g 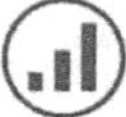

SALMON PATTIES

Ingredients:

- 1 cup steel-cut oats
- ½ cup finely chopped scallions (about 3 scallions)
- 2 tablespoons chopped flat-leaf parsley
- 1 teaspoon kosher salt
- ½ teaspoon freshly ground black pepper
- 2 (14½ oz cans) canned salmon, drained, picked of bones and skin, and flaked
- 2 large eggs, beaten
- 2 tablespoons coarse-grain Dijon mustard
- 6 tablespoons unsalted butter, divided

Directions:

1. Firstly, Put oats in a food processor.
2. Pulse 4 to 5 times or until coarsely ground. Now add salmon, oats, eggs, scallions, mustard, parsley, salt, and pepper in a bowl.
3. Using your hands, mix until well combined. Form into 8 patties. Melt 3 tablespoons butter in a medium nonstick skillet over medium-high.
4. Place 4 salmon patties in skillet and cook until browned, 3 minutes per side.
5. Repeat with remaining butter and patties.

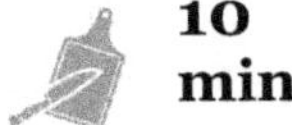 **10 mins** 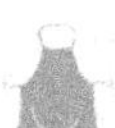 **15 mins** 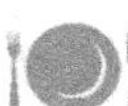 **2/4** 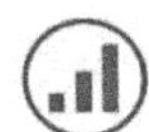 Calories: 245 - Fat: 3,6g - Fiber: 4g
Carbs: 56,9g - Protein: 6g

SEAFOOD STEW

Ingredients:

- 1 tablespoon (½ fl oz – 15 ml) oil
- 6 garlic cloves, minced
- 1 teaspoon kosher salt
- 1 cup (8 fl oz – 240 ml) dry white wine
- 1 large onion, diced
- 1 bay leaf
- 1 (28 oz) can diced tomatoes
- ½ lb. clams
- ½ lb. shrimp, peeled and deveined
- ½ lb. shrimp, peeled and deveined
- 1 cup clam juice
- ½ lb. mussels
- 1/4 cup minced parsley, for garnish, optional

Directions:

1. Take a large pot, heat oil by using medium heat.
2. Put the onions and cook for 3-4 minutes, until tender.
3. Add garlic and sauté for another minute. Now, add the wine, tomatoes, clam juice, bay leaf, and salt. Bring to a boil, then reduce heat to medium and simmer for 20 minutes.
4. Further, put in all the seafood at once and stir to combine.
5. Cook until shrimp is pink and cooked through and mussels and clams have opened about 5-7 minutes. Finely, Garnish with parsley if desired and serve immediately

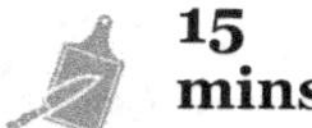 **15 mins**   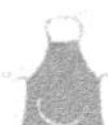 **40 mins**   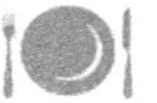 2    Calories: 255 - Fat: 3,1g - Fiber: 5g
Carbs: 65g - Protein: 7g

PRAWN ARRABBIATA

Ingredients:

- 5 oz (125-150 g) Raw or cooked prawns (Ideally king prawns)
- 2 ½ oz (65g) Buckwheat pasta
- 1 tbsp (½ fl oz – 15 ml) Extra virgin olive oil

For arrabbiata sauce

- 1½ oz (40 g) Red onion, finely chopped
- 1 Garlic clove, finely chopped
- 1 oz (30 g) Celery, finely chopped
- 1 Bird's eye chili, finely chopped
- 1 tsp Dried mixed herbs
- 1 tsp (½ fl oz – 15 ml) Extra virgin olive oil
- 2 tbsp (1 fl oz – 30 ml) White wine (optional)
- 14 oz (400 g) Tinned chopped tomatoes
- 1 tbsp Chopped parsley

Directions:

1. Fry the onion, garlic, celery, and chili and dried herbs in the oil over medium-low heat for 1–2 minutes.
2. Turn the heat up to medium, add the wine, and cook for 1 minute. Add the tomatoes and leave the sauce to simmer over medium-low heat for 20–30 minutes, until it has a nice rich consistency.
3. If you feel the sauce is getting too thick, simply add a little water.
4. While the sauce is cooking, bring a pan of water to the boil and cook the pasta according to the packet instructions.
5. When cooked to your liking, drain, toss with the olive oil and keep in the pan until needed.
6. If you are using raw prawns, add them to the sauce and cook for a further3–4 minutes until they have turned pink and opaque, add the parsley and serve.
7. If you are using cooked prawns, add them with the parsley, bring the sauce to the boil and serve.
8. Add the cooked pasta to the sauce, mix thoroughly but gently and serve.

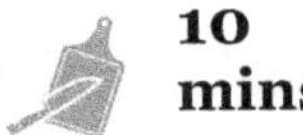 10 mins

 15 mins

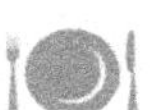 2

Calories: 297 - Fat: 6g - Fiber: 7g
Carbs: 87,5g - Protein: 4,8g

SEARED SALMON WITH CARAMELIZED ENDIVE AND MIXED GREENS

Ingredients:

- 1/3 oz (10 g) parsley
- juice of 1/4 lemon
- 1 clove garlic
- 2 Tablespoon (1 fl oz – 30 ml) extra-virgin olive oil
- 1/4 avocado, stripped, mashed
- 3 ½ oz (100g) cherry tomatoes split
- ¾ oz (20 g) red onion
- 1 ¾ oz (50 g) arugula
- Tablespoons (5 g) celery leaves
- 5 oz (150 g) skinless salmon fillet
- 2 tsp brown sugar
- 1 head of endive

Directions:

1. For the dressing, place the parsley, lemon juice, tricks, garlic, and 2 teaspoons of the oil in a food processor or blender and mix until smooth.
2. For the plate of mixed greens, blend the avocado, tomato, and red onion, arugula, and celery leaves together.
3. Warmth a skillet over high Temperature.
4. Focus on the salmon a little oil and singe it in the hot prospect minute or so to caramelize the outside.
5. Move to a preparing plate and spot in the stove for 5 to 6 minutes or until cooked through; diminish the cooking time by 2 minutes on the off chance that you like your fish served pink inside.
6. In the interim, clear out the skillet and spot it back on high warmth.
7. Blend the earthy colored sugar in with the rest of the teaspoon of oil and brush it over the cut sides of the endive.
8. Spot the endive chop sides down in the hot container and cook for 2 to 3 minutes, turning consistently, until delicate and pleasantly caramelized everywhere.
9. Prepare the plate of mixed greens in the dressing and present with the salmon and endive.

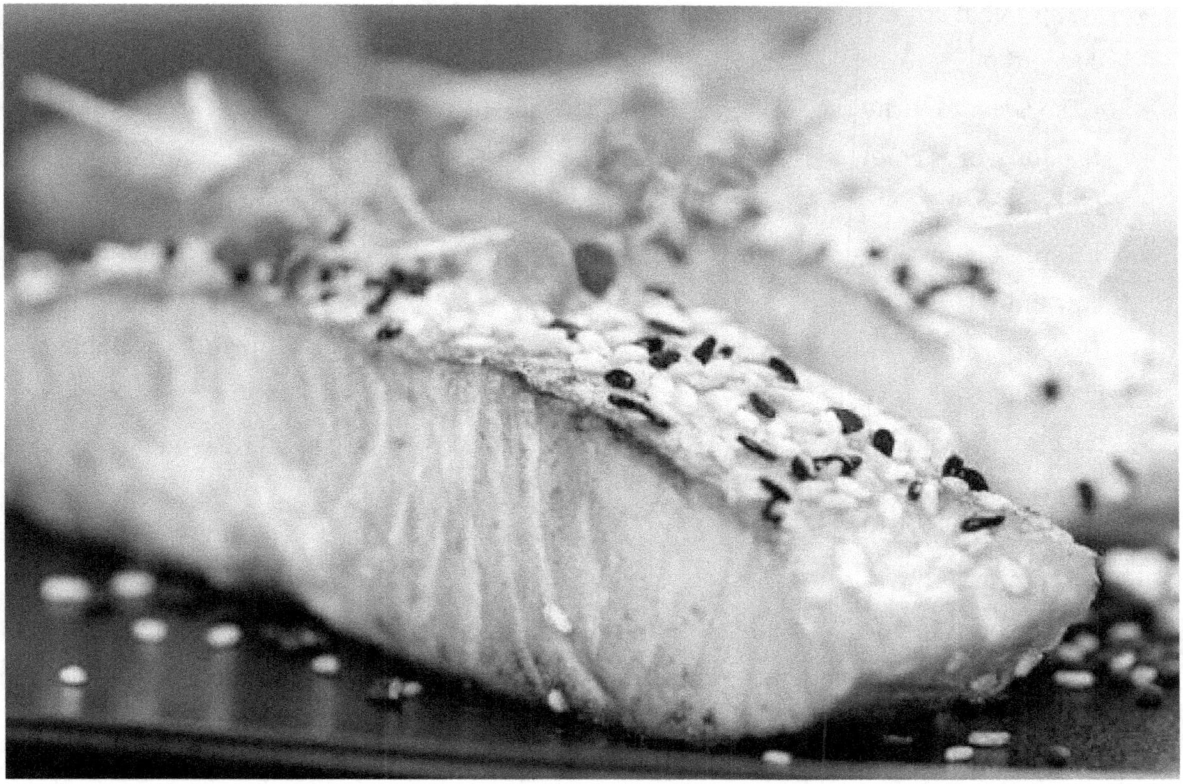

 **10 mins** 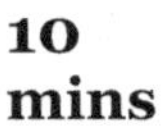 **15 mins** 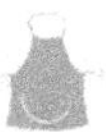 1 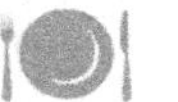 

Calories: 310 - Fat: 7g - Fiber: 6,9g

Carbs: 98g - Protein: 4,8g

TURMERIC BAKED SALMON

Ingredients:

- 5 ½ oz (125-150 g) Skinned Salmon
- 1 Tsp (½ fl oz – 15 ml) extra virgin coconut oil
- 1 Tsp Ground turmeric
- 1/4 Juice of a lemon
- Hot celery:
- 1 Tsp (½ fl oz – 15 ml) extra virgin coconut oil
- 1½ oz (40 g) Red onion, finely chopped
- 2 oz (60 g) Tinned green peas
- 1 Garlic clove, finely chopped
- 0,4 in (1 cm) fresh ginger, finely chopped
- 1 Bird's eye chili, finely chopped
- 5 ½ oz (150 g) Celery, cut into 0,8 in (2cm) lengths
- 1 Tsp curry powder
- 4 ½ oz (130 g) Tomato, cut into 8 wedges
- ½ fl oz (100 ml) vegetable or pasta stock
- 1 tbsp parsley, chopped

Directions:

1. Heat the oven to 200C / gas mark 6. Start using the hot celery.
2. Heat a skillet over a moderate --low heat, then add the olive oil then the garlic, onion, ginger, celery, and peppermint.
3. Fry lightly for two-three minutes until softened but not colored, you can add the curry powder and cook for a further minute. Insert the berries afterward, your lentils and stock, and simmer for 10 seconds.
4. You might choose to increase or reduce the cooking time according to how crunchy you'd like your own sausage.
5. Meanwhile, mix the garlic olive oil and lemon juice and then rub the salmon. # Set on the baking dish and cook 8--10 seconds.
6. To complete, stir the skillet throughout the celery and function with the salmon.

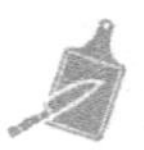 **5 mins**

 **10 mins**

 1

Calories: 288 - Fat: 4,8g - Fiber: 8g
Carbs: 76g - Protein: 5,9g

MALABAR PRAWNS

Ingredients:

- 14 oz (400 g) raw king prawns
- 2 tsp. turmeric
- 3-4 tsp. Kashmiri chili powder
- 4 tsp. (2 fl oz – 60 ml) lemon juice, plus a squeeze
- 1½ oz (40 g) ginger, half peeled and grated, half finely sliced into matchsticks
- 1 tbsp. (½ fl oz – 15 ml) vegetable oil
- 4 curry leaves
- 2-4 green chilies, halved and deseeded
- 1 onion, finely sliced
- 1 tsp. cracked black pepper
- 1½ oz (40 g) fresh coconut, grated
- ½ small bunch coriander leaves only

Directions:

1. Rinse in cool water and pat warm.
2. Connect the turmeric, chili powder, lemon juice, and grated ginger and put aside.
3. Steam oil in a saucepan and incorporate curry leaves, pepper, sliced ginger, and onion.
4. Cook for about 10 minutes, then apply the black pepper.
5. Stir-fry the prawns with some marinade until fried, around 2 minutes.
6. Season if necessary, add lemon juice squeeze.
7. Serve with coconut and coriander leaves.

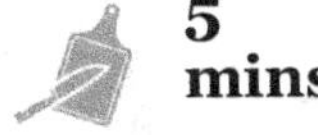 **5 mins** 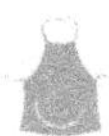 **10 mins** 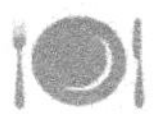 2 Calories: 276 - Fat: 5g - Fiber: 8,1g
Carbs: 78,9g - Protein: 6,9g

VIETNAMESE TURMERIC FISH WITH HERBS & MANGO SAUCE

Ingredients:

- 1 ¼ lb. fresh codfish (skinless and boneless), cut it ½ inch thick and about 2-inch piece wide
- 2 tablespoons (1 fl oz – 30 ml) (plus a few more tablespoon if necessary) coconut oils in a pan and fry the fish
- 1 tablespoon turmeric powder
- 1 teaspoon salt
- 1 tablespoon (½ fl oz – 15 ml) dry sherry or any cooking wine
- 2 tsp minced ginger.
- 2 tbsp (1 fl oz – 30 ml) olive oil
- Scallion and Dill Oil

- 2 cups scallion
- 2 cups fresh doll
- Pinch salt

Mango Dipping sauce

- 1 ripe mango
- 2 tbsp (1 fl oz – 30 ml) rice vinegar
- Juice of lime
- 1 garlic clove
- 1 tsp dry red chili pepper

Toppings:

- Fresh cilantro
- Lime Juice
- Nuts

Directions:

1. Marinate the fish for one hour or as long as it is overnight.
2. Add all ingredients in a mixing bowl under "Mango Dipping Sauce," and combine until quality is obtained.

To Pan-Fry the Fish:

3. Heat 2 tablespoons of coconut oil over the high temperature in a big, nonstick skillet.
4. Add the pre-marinated fish if hot. Note: put the fish slices separately in the saucepan and segregate them into two or more quantities for frying if needed.
5. A loud sizzle should be heard, upon which you can reduce the heat to moderate heat.

6. Do not turn or relocate the fish till after, about 5 minutes, you see a golden-brown skin tone on the side. Top with a tablespoon of sea salt. If required, add more coconut oil to cook the fish.

7. When the fish is in golden brown, move the fish gently on the other side on the cook. Transmit onto a large plate once it's accomplished. Note: The saucepan should have some residual oil in it. We use the remaining oil to make oil that is infused with scallion and dill.

To Make the Scallion and Dill Infused Oil:

8. Just use the rest of the oil over medium to high heat in the frying pan, add 2 cups of scallions, and 2 cups of dill.

9. Remove from the heat once the scallions and dill are introduced. Start giving them a delicate flip, about fifteen seconds, till the scallions and dill simmered.

10. Season with a sprinkle of salt at sea.

11. Plop the scallion, dill, and infused oil over the fish and represent fresh cilantro, lime, and nuts with mango sauce.

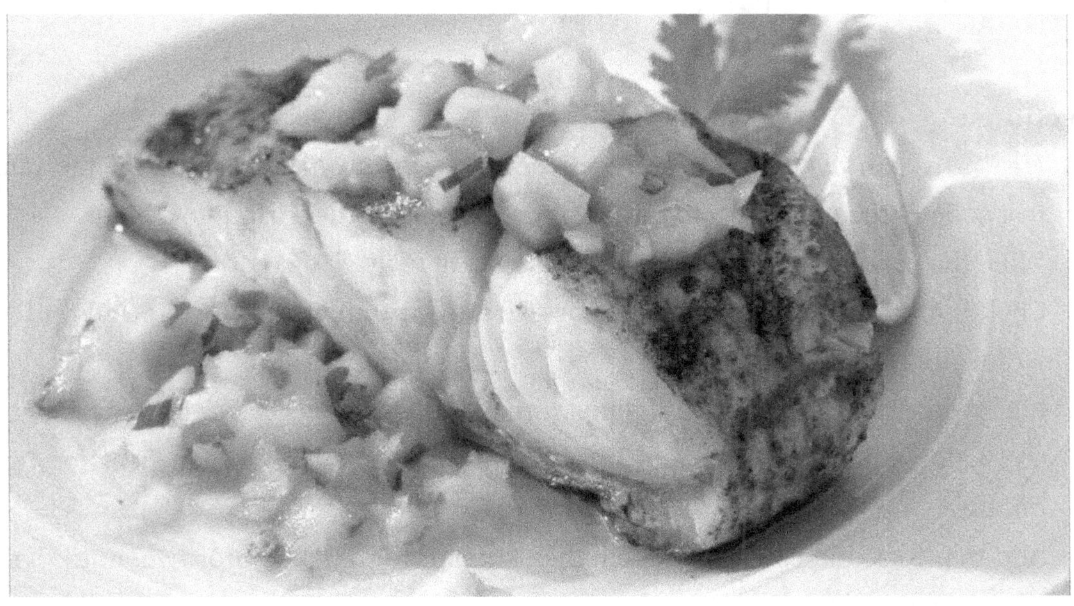

 **30 mins**   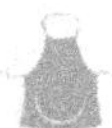 **20 mins**   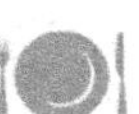 6    Calories: 287 - Fat: 7g - Fiber: 5,9g
Carbs: 80,5g - Protein: 8g

ASIAN SHRIMP STIRFRY

Ingredients:

- 5½ oz (150 g) shelled raw jumbo shrimp, deveined
- 2 teaspoons (¼ fl oz – 10 ml) tamari (or soy, if you're not avoiding gluten)
- 2 teaspoons (¼ fl oz – 10 ml) extra virgin vegetable oil
- 3 oz (75 g) soba (buckwheat noodles)
- 2 garlic cloves, finely chopped
- 1/2 cup (4 fl oz - 120ml) chicken broth
- 1 Thai chili, finely chopped
- 1 teaspoon finely chopped fresh ginger
- ¾ oz (20g) red onions, sliced
- 1 ½ oz (45 g) celery including leaves, trimmed and sliced, with leaves put aside
- 2 ½ oz (75 g) green beans, chopped
- 1 ½ oz (50 g) kale, roughly chopped

Directions:

1. Heat a frypan over high heat, then cook the shrimp in 1 teaspoon of the tamari and 1 teaspoon of the oil for two to three minutes. Transfer the shrimp to a plate.
2. Wipe the pan out with a towel, as you're getting to use it again.
3. Cook the noodles in boiling water for five to eight minutes or as directed on the package. Drain and put aside.
4. Meanwhile, fry the garlic, chili, ginger, red onion, celery (but not the leaves), green beans, and kale within the remaining tamari and oil over medium-high heat for two to three minutes.
5. Add the stock and convey to a boil, then simmer for a moment or two, until the vegetables are cooked but still crunchy.
6. Add the shrimp, noodles, and celery leaves to the pan, bring back to a boil, then remove from the warmth and serve.

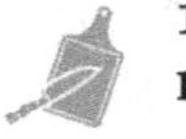 **10 mins** 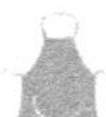 **5 mins**  2  Calories: 286 - Fat: 4,9g - Fiber: 7,8g
Carbs: 79,5g - Protein: 8g

Chapter 11

Main Meals: Pork, Beef, and Lamb

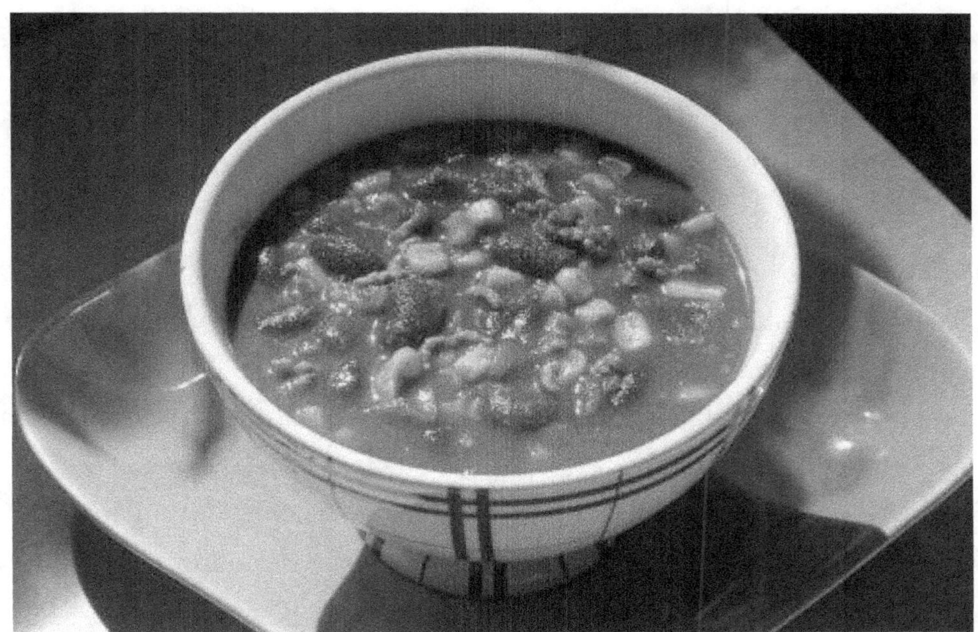

Ingredients:

- 1 ½ lb. (700 g) pork belly
- One tablespoon samba
- 6 cups (50 fl oz – 1,5 liter) of water
- Two tablespoons sugar
- Two tablespoons whole-grain mustard
- 1/2 tablespoon salt
- One teaspoon cayenne
- Three tablespoons (3 fl oz – 90 ml) sherry vinegar
- Two avocados, cubed
- Eight skewers

Directions:

1. Preheat oven to 300°F (150 C°).
2. Place samba, water, sugar, mustard, salt, cayenne, and sherry vinegar in a small saucepan, heat just until sugar and salt dissolve.
3. Place pork in a baking dish and cover with braising liquid. Cover dish with plastic wrap, followed by aluminum foil.
4. Braise in the oven and cook for approximately 3 1/2 hours, or until tender.
5. Remove pork belly and let cool. While the pork belly is cooling, drain liquid and place in a small saucepot.
6. Reduce until consistency has developed, then remove from heat.
7. Once the abdomen is cold, slice into one 1/2-inch cube. Skewer one piece of pork and one piece of avocado on a skewer.
8. Grill while basting with the sauce, and serve.

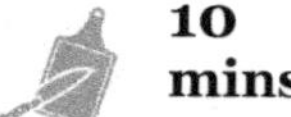 **10 mins** 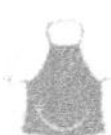 **20 mins** 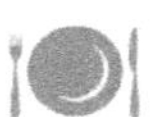 2  Calories: 75 - Fat: 4g - Fiber: 3,4g
Carbs: 54g - Protein: 10,4g

Ingredients:

- 1 lb. (450 g) ground beef
- 1 cup quinoa, rinsed
- ½ cabbage, shredded
- ½ onion, chopped
- 2 leeks, white part only, chopped
- 1 tomato, diced

- 1 tbsp paprika
- ½ tsp cumin
- ½ tsp black pepper
- 4 tbsp extra (2 fl oz – 60 ml) virgin olive oil
- salt, to taste

Directions:

1. In a deep saucepan, sauté the onion and leeks in olive oil until tender.
2. Add in the ground beef, quinoa, tomato, paprika, cumin, salt, and black pepper.
3. Stir very well. Place shredded cabbage on the bottom of an ovenproof baking dish.
4. Cover with beef and quinoa mixture.
5. Cover with a lid or aluminum foil and bake at 325°F (160 C°) for 40 minutes.

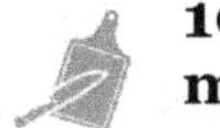 **10 mins** 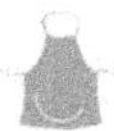 **60 mins** 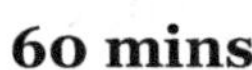 2/3 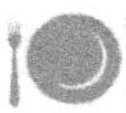 Calories: 245 - Fat: 4,7g - Fiber: 5,8g
Carbs: 67g - Protein: 4,9g

Ingredients:

- 1 Red, finely chopped onion
- Three cloves of garlic, finely chopped
- 2 Thai, finely chopped chilies
- 2 tbsp (1 fl oz – 30 ml) extra virgin olive oil
- 1 Teaspoon cumin in the forest
- 1 Tablespoon of turmeric soil
- 1,6 lb. (725 g) Lean beef (5 % fat)
- red wine (15 fl oz – 450 ml)
- 1 Red bell potato, cored, seeds removed and cut into pieces of bite-size

- Chopped tomatoes 2 x 14 oz (400 g) cans
- 1 Tomato cubit purée
- 1 1/4 cup (10 fl oz - 300ml) canned kidney beef reserve
- 2 Tablespoons (5 g) new, chopped coriander
- 2 Tablespoons (5 g) of fresh, chopped parsley
- 5 ½ oz (160 g) Buckwheat

Directions:

1. Fry the onion, garlic, and chili in the oil for 2 to 3 minutes over medium heat in a big saucepan, then add the spices and fry for another minute or two.
2. Attach the ground beef and cook over medium-high heat for 2 to 3 minutes until the meat is well browned throughout. Add the red wine and allow it to bubble to halve it.
3. Attach the red pepper, onions, purée onions, coffee, kidney beans, and reserve and leave for 1 hour to simmer. Occasionally, you might need to apply a little water to maintain a thick, sticky consistency. Stir in the minced vegetables, right before eating.
4. Furthermore, according to the box directions, cook the buckwheat, and serve with the chili.

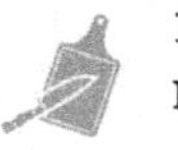 **15 mins**   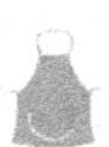 **15/20 mins**    **2/4**    Calories: 310 - Fat: 8g - Fiber: 6g
Carbs: 76g - Protein: 8g

Ingredients:

- 1 gherkin
- 1/3 oz (10 g) of rocket
- 1 oz (30 g) of tomato, sliced
- 5 ½ oz (150 g) of red onion, sliced into rings
- 1/3 oz (10 g) of sliced or grated Cheddar cheese
- 1 unpeeled garlic clove
- 1 tsp of dried rosemary
- 1 tsp (½ fl oz – 15 ml) of olive oil
- 5½ (150 g) of sweet potatoes, peel and cut into 0,4 in (1 cm) thick chips
- 1 tsp (½ fl oz – 15 ml) of olive oil
- 1 tsp of finely chopped parsley
- ½ oz (15 g) of finely chopped red onion
- 4½ oz (125 g) of lean minced beef (5% fat)

Directions:

1. Preheat the oven to 450 f. Toss sweet potato chips with the oil, garlic clove, and rosemary. Add to the baking pan and roast in the oven until nice and crispy, about 30 minutes.
2. Mix the minced beef with parsley and onion. Mold using your hands into an even patty or use a pastry cutter and mold, if you have one.
3. Heat the olive oil over medium heat in a hot frying pan; add onion rings towards one side of the frying pan and the burger over the other.
4. Cook onion rings to your liking and burger for about 6 minutes per side until burger is cooked through.
5. Top the burger with the red onion and cheese, transfer to the preheated oven until cheese is melted. Remove from the oven and top with the tomato, gherkin, and rocket. Serve along with the fries.

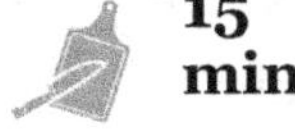 **15 mins**

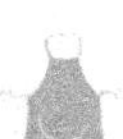 **10 mins**

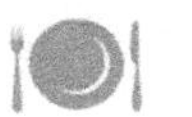 1

 Calories: 345 - Fat: 8,6g - Fiber: 6,4g
Carbs: 76g - Protein: 9,4g

Ingredients:

- 3 oz (75 g) Cous-cous
- 1/2 chicken stock block, composed to 4 ½ fl oz (125 ml)
- 1 oz (30g) pack refreshing flat-leaf parsley, sliced
- 3 mint sprigs, leaves picked and sliced
- 1 tablespoon (½ fl oz – 15 ml) olive oil
- 7 oz (200 g) pack suspended BBQ minted lamb leg beans, De-frosted
- 7 oz (200 g) salad tomatoes, chopped
- 1 spring onion, sliced
- pinch of ground cumin
- 1/2 lemon, zested and juiced
- 2 oz (50 g) reduced-fat salad cheese

Directions:

1. Place the couscous in a heatproof bowl and pour it over the broth.
2. Cover and set aside for 10 minutes, then dust with a fork and mix the herbs.
3. Meanwhile, rub a little oil on the lamb steaks and season. Cook to pack instructions, then slice.
4. Mix the tomatoes, and onion in the couscous with the remaining oil, cumin, lemon zest and juice.
5. Crumble cheese over the salad and serve with the lamb.

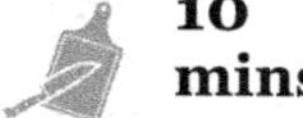 **10 mins**    **10/15 mins**   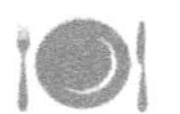 1    Calories: 310 - Fat: 4,9g - Fiber: 8g
Carbs: 56g - Protein: 7g

Ingredients:

- 4 cups (32 ½ fl oz – 950 ml) Beef broth
- 28 oz Fire-roasted crushed tomatoes
- 1 lb. (450 g) Ground beef
- Celery, chopped, 2 stalks
- 1 Onion, diced
- 1 Carrot, chopped
- 1 Bell pepper, diced

- 3 cloves Garlic, minced
- Red cabbage, chopped – 1 head
- 1,5 tbsp Sea salt
- 1 tbsp Italian herb seasoning
- Fresh thyme – 2 sprigs
- 1 tbsp Spicy brown mustard
- 1/8 tsp Black pepper, ground

Directions:

1. Add the ground beef to a large steel soup pot and brown it over medium-high heat until fully cooked. Once done cooking, drain off most of the excess fat, leaving only about two tablespoons in the pot. Set the ground beef aside.

2. Into the now empty soup pot, add the reserved beef fat along with the carrot, celery, onion, and bell pepper. Cook until the vegetables are tender, about six minutes. Add in the garlic and cook until fragrant, about one more minute.

3. Return the cooked ground beef to the soup pot along with the beef broth, crushed tomatoes, seasonings, and spicy brown mustard, stirring it all together to combine.

4. Bring the pot of beef and tomatoes to a boil and then reduce to a simmer, cooking for fifteen to twenty minutes.

5. Stir the cabbage into the soup, allowing it to cook until tender, about ten to fifteen minutes. Serve alone or over either cooked rice or buckwheat.

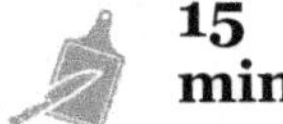 **15 mins** 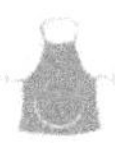 **25/30 mins** 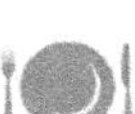 **2/4** Calories: 320 - Fat: 5,8g - Fiber: 4,6g
Carbs: 68g - Protein: 8g

Chapter 12

Main Meals: Poultry

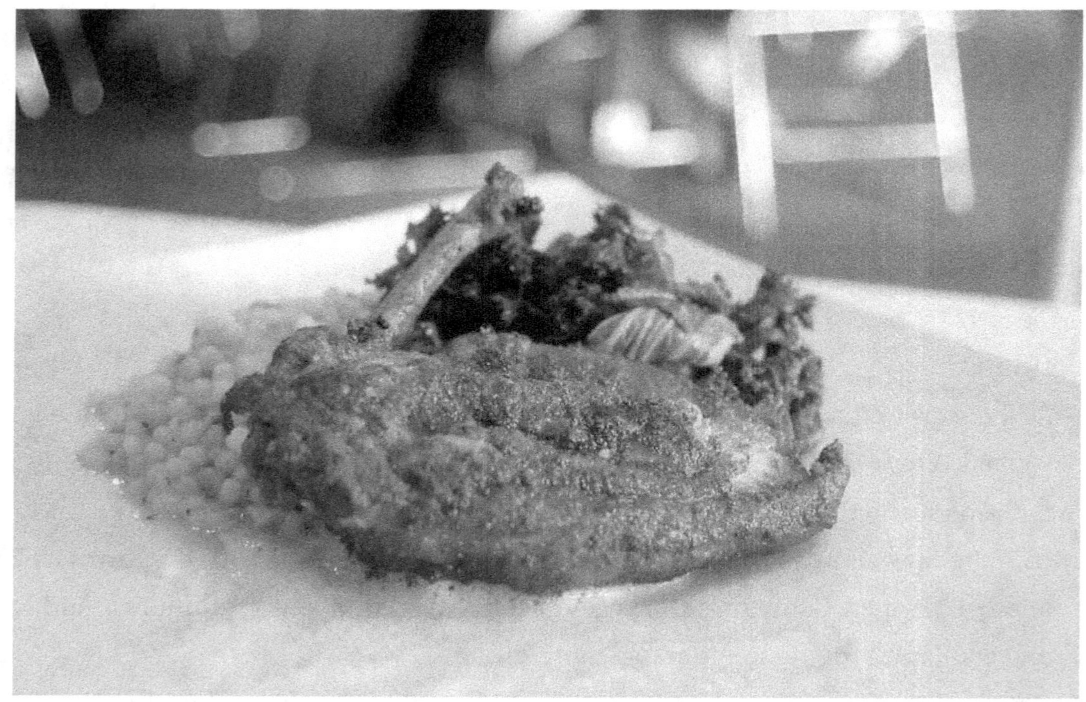

Ingredients:

- 9 oz (250 g) tinned chickpeas garbanzo beans drained
- 4 chicken breasts, cubed
- 4 Medrol dates halved
- 6 dried apricots, halved
- 1 red onion, sliced
- 1 carrot, chopped
- 2 fl oz (60 ml) water

- 1 teaspoon ground cumin
- 1 teaspoon ground cinnamon
- 1 teaspoon ground turmeric
- 1 bird's-eye chili, chopped
- 120 fl oz (600 ml) chicken stock broth
- 1 oz (25 g) cornflour
- 2 tablespoons fresh coriander

Directions:

1. Place the chicken, chickpeas garbanzo beans, onion, carrot, chili, cumin, turmeric, cinnamon, and stock broth into a large saucepan.
2. Put it to the boil, and reduce heat after that simmer for 25 minutes.
3. Add in the dates and apricots and simmer for 10 minutes. In a cup, mix the cornflour together with the water until it becomes a smooth paste.
4. Pour the mixture into the saucepan and stir until it thickens.
5. Add in the coriander cilantro and mix well. Serve with buckwheat or couscous.

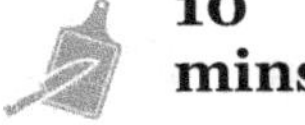 **10 mins** 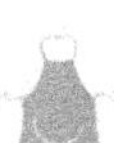 **15/30 mins** 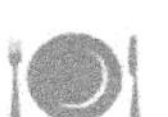 2  Calories: 230 - Fat: 3,8g - Fiber: 6,5g
Carbs: 69,8g - Protein: 8g

Ingredients:

- 1 tbsp (½ fl oz – 15 ml) groundnut oil or sunflower oil
- 12 oz (340 g) pack of mini chicken breast fillets
- 6 ½ (200 ml) chicken stock
- lemon Zest or juice
- 7 oz (200 g) pack tender stem broccoli
- 1 tsp heaped cornflour
- 2 garlic cloves, sliced
- 2 tsp golden caster sugar
- a handful of roasted cashews

Directions:

1. Take a large frypan and preheat the oil for 2-3 minutes.
2. Put the chicken and fry for almost 3-4 minutes until it turns golden.
3. Remove the chicken from the pan and now add the garlic cloves and broccoli.
4. Stir fry for a minute or so than covers and cook for almost 2 minutes more until it becomes tender.
5. After that, mix the stock, cornflour, and sugar well, then pour into the pan and stir until it becomes thickened.
6. Now, add the chicken back into the pan and let it cook through, then mix the lemon zest and juice, and cashew nuts.
7. Stir, then serve immediately with rice or noodles.

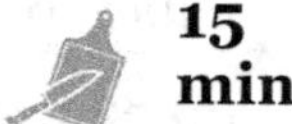 **15 mins**  **20/25 mins** 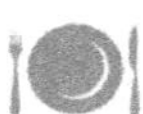 2  Calories: 275 - Fat: 3,8g - Fiber: 7g
Carbs: 67g - Protein: 6g

Ingredients:

- 1 tablespoon (½ fl oz – 15 ml) sunflower oil
- 26 ½ oz (750 g) package chicken thighs, boned, any surplus skin trimmed
- 9 oz (250 g) frozen chopped mixed peppers
- 1 Inch courgette, peeled into ribbons, seeded center chopped
- 1 chicken stock cube
- 9 oz (250 g) egg yolks
- 4 garlic cloves, finely chopped
- 1/2 tsp crushed chilies, and additional to serve (optional)
- 4 tablespoons (1 fl oz – 30 ml) reduced-salt soy sauce
- 2 tsp caster sugar
- 1 lime, zested, 1/2 juiced, 1/2 slice into wedges to function

Directions:

1. Heat the oil in a skillet on a medium-low warmth. Fry the chicken skin-side down to 10 mins or until your skin is emptied. Flip and simmer for 10 mins, or until cooked.
2. Transfer to a plate cover loosely with foil.
3. Reheat the wok over a high temperature, add the peppers and sliced courgette; simmer for 5 mins. Meanwhile, bring a bowl of water to the boil, then crumble in the stock block, adding the noodles. Simmer for 45 mins until cooked, then drain well.
4. Insert the garlic and crushed chilies into the wok; simmer for two mins. In a bowl, mix the soy sugar and the lime juice and zest. Enhance the wok, bubble 2 mins; you can add the courgette noodles and ribbons. Toss with tongs to coat in the sauce.
5. Cut the chicken into pieces. Divide the noodles between 4 bowls and top with the chicken. Serve with the lime wedges along with extra crushed chilies, in case you prefer.

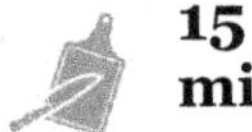 **15 mins** 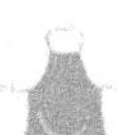 **20 mins** 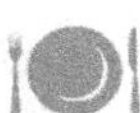 **2/4**  Calories: 287 - Fat: 4,7g - Fiber: 6,2g
Carbs: 59,9g - Protein: 8,5g

Ingredients:

- 12 oz (350 g) spaghetti
- 1 cup cooked chicken, shredded
- 2 avocados, peeled and diced
- 1 cup cherry tomatoes, halved
- 1 garlic clove, chopped
- 2 tbsp basil pesto
- 5 tbsp (2 ½ fl oz – 75 ml) olive oil
- 4 tbsp (2 fl oz – 60 ml) lemon juice
- ¼ cup grated parmesan cheese

Directions:

1. In a large pot of boiling salted water, cook spaghetti according to package directions. Drain and set aside in a large bowl.
2. In a blender, combine lemon juice, garlic, basil pesto, and avocados and blend until smooth.
3. Combine spaghetti, chicken, cherry tomatoes, and avocado sauce.
4. Sprinkle with parmesan cheese and serve immediately.

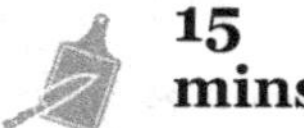 15 mins 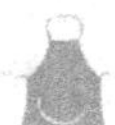 15 mins  2 

Calories: 285 - Fat: 4,3g - Fiber: 6g

Carbs: 56g - Protein: 8,5g

Ingredients:

- 2 teaspoons minced garlic
- 1 tablespoon crunchy nutty spread (change in accordance together with your preferences)
- 2 tablespoons earthy colored sugar, stuffed
- Salt to season
- 1 cup (8 fl oz – 250 ml) light coconut milk
- 1 teaspoon turmeric
- 3 tablespoons powdered nutty spread
- 21 oz (600 g) turkey bosom filets, cubed
- Extra water if necessary
- Fresh coriander leaves
- 12 wooden sticks
- Coconut oil splash

Directions:

1. Put turkey pieces on sticks and chill it for 30 minutes. Mic all ingredients in a bowl and mix well.
2. Add marinade to turkey sticks for a few hours or even overnight. After marinating, drain the marinade from the turkey and on a pan, heat oil, add turkey sticks and cook over medium heat for around 4 -5 minutes each side.
3. Flip and cook thoroughly with some marinade for more minutes until fully cooked. For the remaining marinade, heat the excess in a saucepan for about 5 minutes.
4. Add water if it becomes too thick. Pour over turkey sticks.
5. Serve sticks with leaves of coriander, steamed rice or vegetables, and sprinkle with satay sauce.

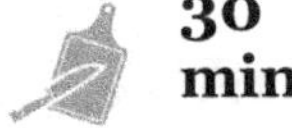 **30 mins**  **15/20 mins** 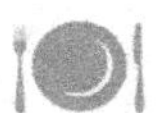 2 Calories: 276 - Fat: 4g - Fiber: 6,1g
Carbs: 45g - Protein: 4,9g

FRIED CHICKEN AND BROCCOLINI

Ingredients:

- 2 tablespoon (1 fl oz – 30 ml) Coconut oil
- 14 oz (400 g) Chicken breast
- 5 ½ oz (150 g) Bacon cubes
- 9 oz (250 g) Broccolini

Directions:

1. Cut the chicken into cubes.
2. Melt the coconut oil in a pan over medium heat and brown the chicken with the bacon cubes and cook through.
3. Season with chili flakes, salt, and pepper.
4. Add broccolini and fry. Stack on a plate and enjoy!

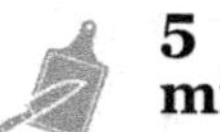 5 mins

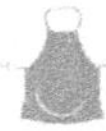 10 mins

 1

Calories: 187 - Fat: 2,4g - Fiber: 3,1g

Carbs: 34,5g - Protein: 4g

TURKEY ESCALOPES WITH SPICED CAULIFLOWER "COUSCOUS"

Ingredients:

- 5 ½ oz (150 g) cauliflower, roughly chopped
- 2 garlic cloves, finely chopped
- 1 ½ oz (40 g) purple onion, finely chopped
- 1 Thai chili, finely chopped
- 1 teaspoon finely chopped fresh ginger
- 2 tablespoons (1 fl oz – 30 ml) extra virgin vegetable oil
- 2 teaspoons ground turmeric
- 1 oz (30 g) sun-dried tomatoes, finely chopped
- 1/3 oz (10 g) fresh parsley, chopped
- 5 ½ (150 g) turkey cutlet or steak
- 1/8 fl oz dried sage juice of 1/4 lemon
- 1 tablespoon capers

Directions:

1. To make the "couscous," place the raw cauliflower during a kitchen appliance.
2. Pulse in 2-second bursts to finely chop the cauliflower until it resembles couscous. Alternatively, you'll just use a knife and chop it very finely.
3. Fry the garlic, red onion, chili, and ginger in 1 teaspoon of the oil until soft but not browned.
4. Add the turmeric and cauliflower and cook for 1 minute.
5. Remove from heat and add the sun-dried tomatoes and half the parsley.
6. Coat the turkey escalope within the sage and a touch oil, then use the remaining oil to fry during a frypan over medium heat for five to six minutes, turning regularly.
7. When cooked through, add the juice, remaining parsley, capers, and 1 tablespoon of water to the pan.
8. This may create a sauce to serve with the cauliflower.

 **15 mins**   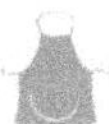 **10 mins**   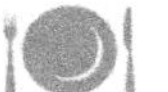 1   .il   Calories: 290 - Fat: 4,3g - Fiber: 6g
Carbs: 47g - Protein: 8g

CHICKEN BREAST IN TOMATO SALSA WITH KALE AND RED ONIONS

Ingredients:

- 4 ½ oz (12 0g) skinless, boneless chicken bosom
- 2 teaspoons ground turmeric
- juice of 1/4 lemon
- 1 tablespoon (1/2 fl oz – 15ml) extra-virgin olive oil
- 1 ½ oz (50 g) kale, slashed
- 1/3 oz (20 g) red onion, cut

- 1 teaspoon slashed new ginger
- 1 ½ oz (50 g) buckwheat

FOR THE SALSA

- 1 medium tomato (4 ½ oz – 130 g)
- 1 Thai beans, blanched
- 2 tablespoons (5 g) parsley,
- juice of 1/4 lemon

Directions:

1. Blend in with the stew, tricks, parsley, and lemon juice. You could place everything in a blender; however, the final product is somewhat extraordinary.
2. Marinate the chicken bosom in 1 teaspoon of the turmeric, the lemon juice, and a little oil. Leave for 5 to 10 minutes.
3. Warmth an ovenproof griddle until hot, at that point include the marinated chicken and cook for a moment or so on each side, until pale brilliant, at that point move to the broiler (place on a preparing plate if your dish isn't ovenproof) for 8 to 10 minutes or until cooked through.
4. Expel from the broiler, spread with foil, and leave to rest for 5 minutes before serving.
5. In the interim, cook the kale in a liner for 5 minutes.
6. Fry the red onions and the ginger in a little oil, until delicate yet not seared, at that point include the cooked kale and fry for one more moment.
7. Cook the buckwheat as indicated by the bundle directions with the rest of the teaspoon of turmeric. Serve nearby the chicken, vegetables, and salsa.

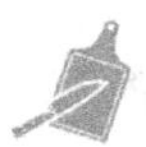 **10 mins** 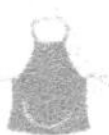 **15/20 mins** 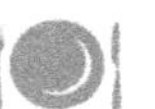 1 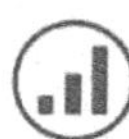 Calories: 289 - Fat: 3,5g - Fiber: 5,3g
Carbs: 45g - Protein: 7g

BAKED POTATOES WITH SPICY CHICKPEA STEW

Ingredients:

- 4-6 baking potatoes, pricked all over,
- 1 fl oz (30 ml) olive oil,
- 2 red onions, finely chopped,
- 4 cloves garlic, grated or crushed,
- 0,8 in (2cm) ginger, grated,
- ½ -2 teaspoons chili flakes (depending on how hot you like things),
- 2 tablespoons cumin seeds,
- 2 tablespoons turmeric,
- Splash of water,
- 2 x 14 oz (400 g) tins chopped tomatoes,
- 2 tablespoons unsweetened cocoa powder (or cacao),
- 2 yellow peppers (or whatever color you prefer!), cut into bite-size pieces,
- 2 spoonfuls of parsley plus extra to garnish Salt and pepper (optional), side salad (optional),

Directions:

1. Preheat the oven to 400° F; all of your ingredients can be prepared by now. Place potatoes in the oven when the oven is hot enough, and cook them for 1 hour or until they're finished as you like them.
2. Put the olive oil and chopped red onion in a very broad saucepan once the potatoes are in the oven and cook gently, with the lid on for 5 minutes, until the onions are soft but not brown. Remove the cover and add the garlic, cumin, ginger, and chili.
3. Cook over low heat for another minute, then add the turmeric and a very tiny splash of water and cook for another minute, taking care not to warm the pan.
4. Next, add cocoa powder (or cacao), chickpeas (including chickpea water) and yellow pepper to the tomatoes.
5. Bring to boil and cook for 45 minutes at low heat until the sauce is thick and greasy (but don't let it burn!).
6. The stew should be handled roughly at the same time as the potatoes.

7. Finally, stir in the two parsley tablespoons and, if you wish, some salt and pepper, and serve the stew on top of the baked potatoes, perhaps with a simple side salad.

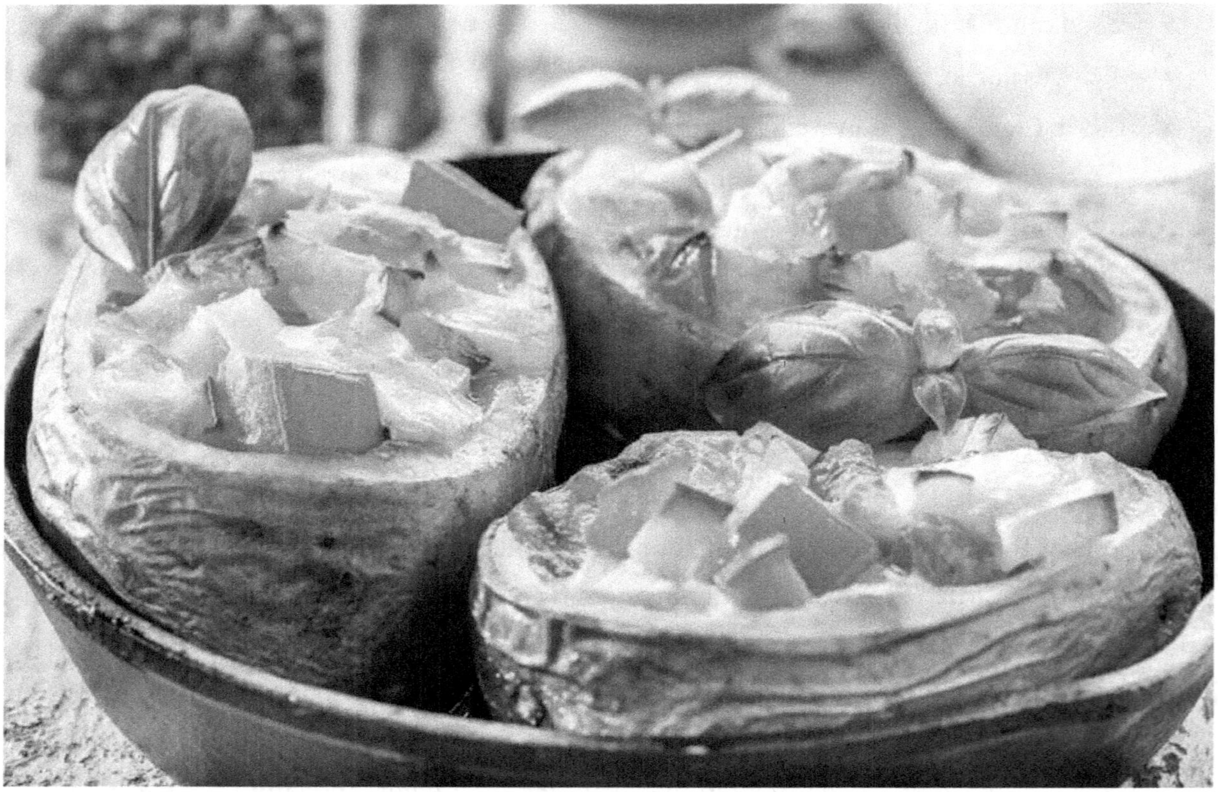

10 mins

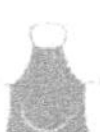
45/50 mins

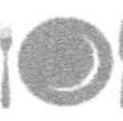
2/4

Calories: 315 - Fat: 5g - Fiber: 6,8g
Carbs: 60g - Protein: 6g

CHICKEN AND CHICKPEA FRITTERS

Ingredients:

- 1 can chickpeas, drained
- 2 chicken breasts, cooked and shredded
- 2 egg whites
- 1 tsp ginger
- ½ cup fresh parsley leaves, very finely cut
- ½ tsp black pepper salt, to taste
- 2 tbsp (1 fl oz – 30 ml) coconut oil, for frying

Directions:

1. Blend the chickpeas in a food processor and combine them with the chicken, egg whites, parsley, and ginger into a smooth batter.
2. Heat the oil in a frying pan over medium heat.
3. Using a large tbsp, form the batter into fritters.
4. Cook each one for 2-3 minutes each side or until golden and cooked through.

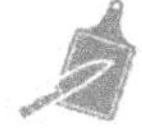 5 mins 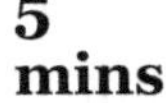 15 mins 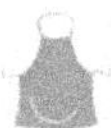 2 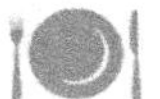

Calories: 175 - Fat: 2,8g - Fiber: 4,3g
Carbs: 35g - Protein: 6,1g

Chapter 13

Main Meals: Non-meat

BALSAMIC ROASTED CARROTS AND BABY ONIONS

Ingredients:

- 2 bunches baby carrots, scrubbed, ends trimmed
- 10 small onions, peeled, halved
- 4 tbsp brown sugar
- 1 tsp thyme
- 2 tbsp (1 fl oz – 30 ml) extra virgin olive oil

Directions:

1. Preheat oven to 350°F (180 C°).
2. Line a baking tray with baking paper. Place the carrots, onions, thyme, and oil in a large bowl and toss until well coated.
3. Arrange carrots and onions, in a single layer, on the baking tray.
4. Roast for 20 minutes or until tender. Sprinkle over the sugar and vinegar and toss to coat.
5. Roast for 20 minutes more or until the vegetables are tender and caramelized.
6. Season with salt and pepper to taste and serve.

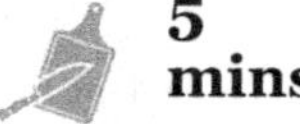 **5 mins** 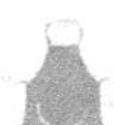 **30 mins** 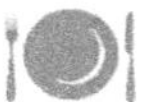 2 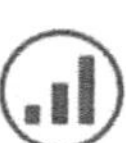 Calories: 200 - Fat: 3g - Fiber: 4,1g
Carbs: 35g - Protein: 6,4g

Ingredients:

- 1 can chickpeas, drained and rinsed
- 1 small carrot, cut
- 1 onion, cut
- 2 garlic cloves, minced
- ½ cup fresh parsley, finely cut
- ¼ cup whole wheat flour

- ¼ cup tahini
- 2 fl oz (60 ml) extra virgin olive oil
- 1 ½ fl oz (50 ml) lemon juice
- 2 tsp cumin (or to taste)
- 1 tsp salt
- Black pepper, to taste

Directions:

1. Blend the carrots, chickpeas, onion, and garlic in a food processor until completely minced.
2. When it turns to a smooth paste, add in parsley and transfer to a large mixing bowl.
3. Stir in the remaining ingredients.
4. Using a large tbsp form batter into burgers.
5. Bake in a preheated to 375°F (190° C) oven until golden.

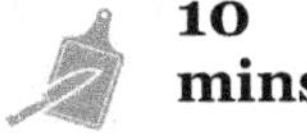 **10 mins**   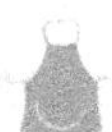 **20 mins**   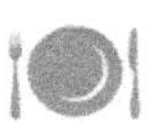 **2**   Calories: 276 - Fat: 5g - Fiber: 7g
Carbs: 65g - Protein: 8g

Ingredients:

- 14 oz Tofu, firm
- 8 tablespoons Cornstarch, divided
- 1 Egg white
- 1 cup Pineapple, chopped
- 2 Bell pepper, chopped
- 3 fl oz (100 ml) Rice vinegar
- 6 tbsp Date sugar
- 1 fl oz (30 ml) Tamari sauce
- 1 tsp Sea salt
- 2 tbsp Tomato paste
- 1/3 fl oz (10 ml) Water
- 2 tbsp Cornstarch
- 1 tsp Sesame seeds, toasted

Directions:

1. Line an aluminum baking sheet with kitchen parchment or a silicone sheet and set the oven to Fahrenheit three-hundred and fifty degrees.
2. Begin by pressing your tofu and then slicing it into bite-sized cubes. Sprinkle two of the eight divided tablespoons of cornstarch over the tofu, tossing it until the tofu is evenly coated.
3. Place the remaining six tablespoons of divided cornstarch in one bowl and the egg white in another. Dip a few tofu cubes at a time first in the egg white and then in the cornstarch. Transfer the breaded cubes to the prepared baking sheet and continue the process until all the cubes are prepared.
4. Arrange the tofu cubes on the pan evenly so that they don't touch, and then bake until crispy, about fifteen to twenty minutes.
5. While the tofu cooks, whisk together the rice vinegar, date sugar, tamari sauce, sea salt, tomato paste, water, two tablespoons of corn starch, and the sesame seeds.
6. Add the peppers and pineapple to a large skillet and sauté them until slightly tender. Add in the mixed sauce and deglaze the skillet.
7. Add the cooked tofu to the skillet and continue to cook it in the sauce until it is coated and sticky, and the sauce has thickened. Serve while warm over brown rice or buckwheat.

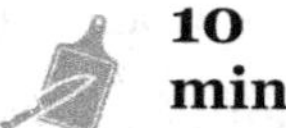 **10 mins**  **25 mins** 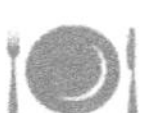 2  Calories: 230 - Fat: 4g - Fiber: 2,7g
Carbs: 48,9g - Protein: 4,3g

Ingredients:

- 14 oz (400 g) Tofu, extra-firm, sliced into bite-sized cubes
- 1 tsp Cumin
- 2 tsp Ginger, peeled and grated
- ½ tsp Sweet paprika
- ½ tsp Turmeric
- 2 cloves Garlic, minced
- ¼ fl oz (8 ml) Garam masala
- ½ tsp Coriander powder
- ¼ tsp Cayenne
- 8 fl oz (250 ml) Tomato passata (if not available use puree)
- 14 fl oz (400 ml) Coconut milk, full-fat
- 1 fl oz (30 ml) Olive oil
- 1 Red onion, diced
- 1 tsp Sea salt

Directions:

1. Add the olive oil, red onion, and salt to a skillet and allow it to cook over medium until the onions have become soft about five minutes.
2. Add in the grated ginger and minced garlic, cooking for a minute before adding in all the spices. Cook for an additional two minutes, until the spices are fragrant.
3. Keep a close eye on the spices, constantly stirring to avoid burning.
4. Stir the tomato passata or puree into the skillet and allow it to continue cooking until thickened and reduced, about ten to fifteen minutes.
5. Add the tofu and canned coconut milk to the skillet and bring the pan to a boil. Reduce the stove to low and allow the tikka masala to simmer for ten minutes. Serve warm over brown rice or buckwheat.

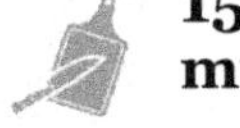 **15 mins** 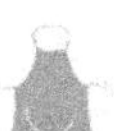 **20 mins** 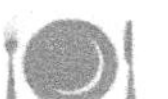 2

Calories: 220 - Fat: 5g - Fiber: 6,8g
Carbs: 45g - Protein: 8g

Ingredients:

- 8 ½ fl oz (250 ml) vegetable stock
- 1 big bunch of asparagus, chopped
- 2 cloves of garlic, minced
- 1 fl oz (30 ml) macadamia, olive, or coconut oil, divided
- 1 small white onion, finely chopped
- 9 oz (250 g) buckwheat, soaked overnight + drained and rinsed
- 1 small white onion, finely chopped
- 1 tablespoon dried Italian herbs
- 4 ½ (120 g peas), fresh or thawed frozen
- Large handful spinach, finely chopped
- Salt + pepper
- 1 lemon, juiced and zested
- A handful of parsley, oregano and basil, roughly chopped + more for topping
- 2 tablespoons nutritional yeast
- Extra virgin olive oil, for drizzling

Directions:

1. Start with preparing veggie stock in a pan and boil them now dim the heat to simmer finely. Take a large pan, heat 1 tbsp of oil and fry your asparagus on light heat, until tender but still retains a bite -around 1 minute.

2. Now, remove from the pan and put it aside. Now, add the remaining oil along with the onion and garlic in the same pan and cook until soft, about 5 minutes.

3. Put the buckwheat, dried herbs, apple cider vinegar, and lemon juice to the pan and stir so that every ingredient is finely coated. After that, put in veggie stock a little bit at a time, occasionally stirring, just like you would ordinary risotto.

4. Once the buckwheat is almost fully cooked, almost 10 minutes in, stir in your peas and spinach.

5. Cook more for few minutes, then turn off the heat, stir in your herbs, lemon zest, nutritional yeast, salt, and pepper.

6. Taste and adjust seasoning, either putting in some more lemon juice or yeast for a cheesier flavor. Use the asparagus, herbs, and olive oil as toppings and serve.

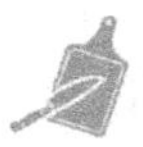 **10 mins** 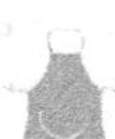 **15/20 mins** 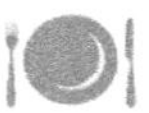 4 Calories: 218 - Fat: 4g - Fiber: 4,3g
Carbs: 37,6g - Protein: 5,7g

Ingredients:

- 12 oz Korean buckwheat noodles
- 1 x 12 oz jar napa kimchi
- 1 tablespoon (or more) sugar
- 1 tablespoon toasted sesame oil
- Salt
- 4 scallions, thinly sliced
- ½ cucumber, julienned
- 2 large eggs, hardboiled, quartered
- ½ cup thinly sliced toasted laver or nori sheets
- 2 tablespoons toasted sesame seeds
- 1 fl oz (30 ml) (or more) rice wine vinegar

Directions:

1. Take a large pot of water and boil it. Put noodles and cook, occasionally stirring, until cooked through, but still slightly bouncy, about 1½ minutes.
2. Now, Drain and rinse under cold running water; put it aside.
3. Drain kimchi, reserving liquid; chop the kimchi. Combine kimchi, kimchi liquid, vinegar, oil, and sugar in a large bowl and toss to combine.
4. Next, add the cooked noodles and toss to coat; season with salt and more vinegar or sugar.
5. Serve the dish with egg, cucumber, scallions, laver, sesame seeds, and 2 cups crushed ice.

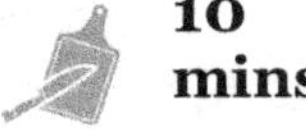 **10 mins** 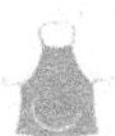 **15 mins** 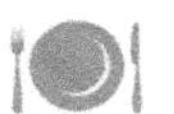 **2**

Calories: 189 - Fat: 2,5g - Fiber: 3,2g
Carbs: 30g - Protein: 6g

Ingredients:

- A small bunch of dill, chopped
- Salt and freshly ground black pepper
- 9 oz (250 g) of brown mushrooms
- 1 tbsp (1/2 fl oz – 15 ml) of olive oil
- A small bunch of parsley, less than dill, chopped
- 2 tbsp of butter, divided
- 3 small red onions, thinly sliced
- 15 fl oz (450 ml) of chicken stock or vegetable broth (a bit less than 16 fl oz - 500 ml)
- 1 egg
- 5½ oz (150 g) of roasted buckwheat groats

Directions:

1. Lightly whisk the egg in a bowl. Mix in the buckwheat until well mixed.
2. Heat a non-stick pan over medium heat, add buckwheat and cook until all the corns are separated and dry about 3-4 minutes.
3. Transfer the buckwheat to a small saucepan. Add in the stock or broth and bring to a boil, reduce heat, and let it simmer for 15 minutes or thereabout until the stock has been absorbed and the buckwheat is soft. Heat the olive oil with 1 tbsp.
4. Butter in the pan on low heat; add onions and cook, often stirring for 15 minutes or until tender and golden brown. You can add a few splashes of water in between so the onion won't catch.
5. Add in the mushrooms and cook for additional 5-7 minutes or until withered and cooked; season with salt and pepper.
6. Add in buckwheat and stir to coat well. Stir in the remaining butter. Add in chopped parsley and dill.
7. Serve with some green salad.

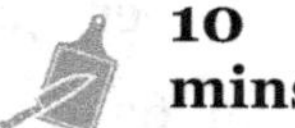 **10 mins**

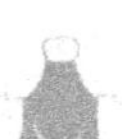 **10/15 mins**

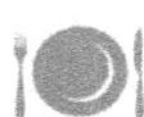 2

Calories: 220 - Fat: 3,6g - Fiber: 5,5g
Carbs: 39g - Protein: 7g

Ingredients:

- 1 Tablespoon (1/2 fl oz – 30 ml) Virgin Olive Oil
- 1 ½ oz (50 g) red onion
- 1 oz (30 g) carrot, strips
- 1 oz (30 g) celery
- Garlic Cloves
- 1/2 Thai stew
- 1 teaspoon herbs de Provence
- 7/8 fl oz (200 ml) vegetable stock
- 1 x 14-oz can (400 g) Italian tomatoes
- 1 teaspoon tomato purée
- 4 ½ oz (130 g) canned blend beans
- 1 ½ oz (50 g) kale, generally hacked
- 1 tablespoon parsley
- 1 ½ oz (50 g) buckwheat

Directions:

1. Spot the oil in a medium pot over low to medium warmth and delicately fry the onion, carrot, celery, garlic, bean stew (if utilizing), and herbs, until the onion is delicate however not sautéed.

2. Include the stock, tomatoes, and tomato purée and heat to the point of boiling. Include the beans and stew for 30 minutes.

3. Include the kale and cook for another 5 to 10 minutes until delicate, at that point, include the parsley.

4. In the interim, cook the buckwheat as per the bundle directions, channel, and afterward present with the stew.

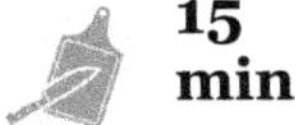 **15 mins**  **40 mins**  2 

Calories: 298 - Fat: 6g - Fiber: 5,8g
Carbs: 54g - Protein: 4,9g

HARISSA BAKED TOFU WITH CAULIFLOWER COUSCOUS

Ingredients:

- 2 oz (60 g) red bell pepper
- 1 Thai chili halved
- 2 garlic cloves
- about 1 tablespoon (1/2 fl oz – 30 ml) of extra virgin olive oil
- pinch of ground cumin
- pinch of ground coriander
- juice of ¼ lemon
- 7 oz (200 g) rm tofu

- 7 oz (200 g) cauliflower, roughly chopped
- 1½ oz (40 g) red onion, finely chopped
- 1 teaspoon of nicely chopped fresh ginger
- 1 oz (30 g) of sun-dried tomatoes, finely chopped
- 1 /3 oz (20 g) of parsley, chopped

Directions:

1. Heat the oven to 400°F (200°C).
2. Slice the red pepper lengthwise around the center to make the harissa, so you have nice slices, remove any seeds, then put the chili and one of the garlic cloves in a roasting pan.
3. Add a little oil and the dried cumin and coriander and roast for 15 to 20 minutes in the oven until the peppers are soft but not too hot. (Leave the oven on at this setting.)
4. Cool, then mix with the lemon juice into a food processor until smooth.
5. Lengthwise slice the tofu and then diagonally cut into triangles every half.
6. Place in a small non-stick roasting pan or one lined with parchment paper, cover with harissa, and roast for 20 minutes in the oven — the tofu would have absorbed the marinade and turned dark red.
7. Place the raw cauliflower in a food processor to produce the "couscous" Pulse to finely chop the cauliflower in 2-second bursts until it resembles couscous. Alternatively, just use a knife and neatly cut it.

8. Thin out the remaining clove of garlic. In 1 teaspoon of oil, fry the garlic, red onion and ginger, until soft but not browned, then add the turmeric and cauliflower and cook for 1 minute.

9. Remove from heat and mix in the tomatoes and parsley, which are dried with light. Serve with the tofu, which is baked.

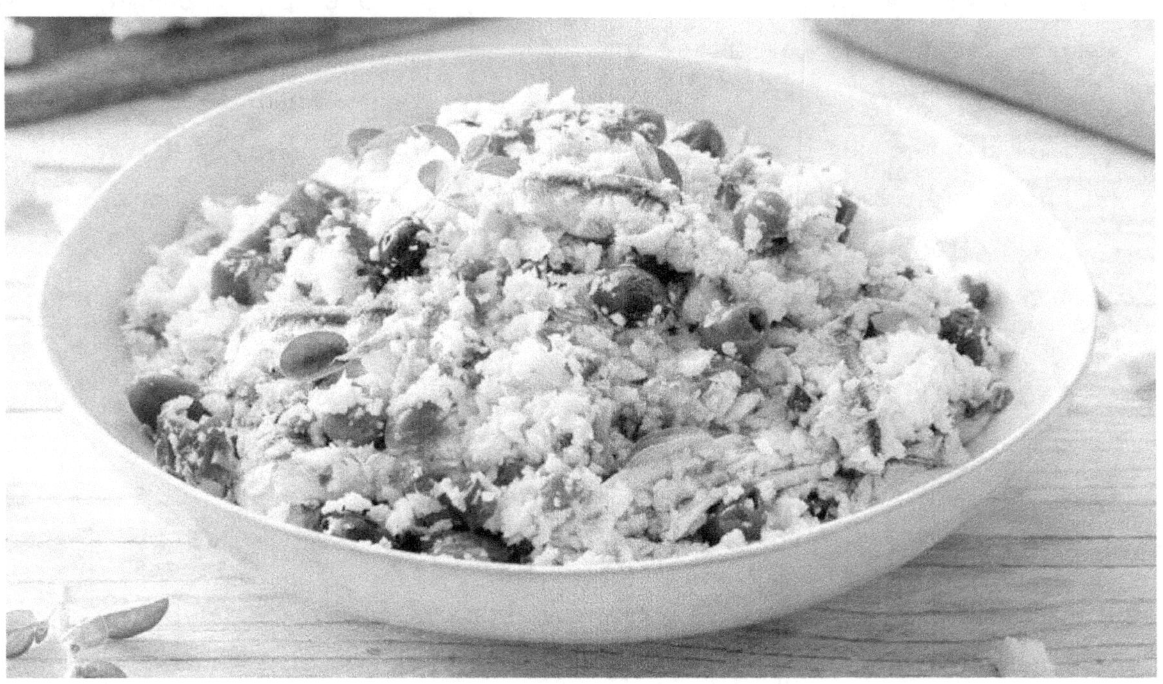

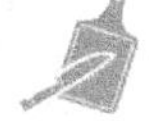 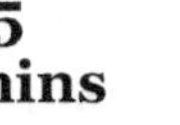 **15 mins** 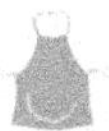 **40 mins** 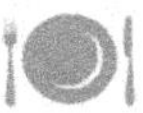 2 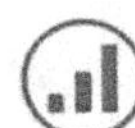 Calories: 199 - Fat: 2,9g - Fiber: 5g
Carbs: 41g - Protein: 7,4g

Ingredients:

- 2 wood skewers, soaked in water for 30 minutes before use.
- 8 large black olives.
- 8 cherry tomatoes.
- 1 yellow pepper, cut into eight squares.
- 1/2 red onion, halved and separated into eight pieces.
- 3 ½ oz (100 g) (about 4 in - 10 cm) cucumber, cut into four slices and halved.
- 3 ½ oz (100 g) feta, cut into eight cubes.

- For the dressing:
- One tablespoon extra virgin olive oil.
- Juice of 1/2 lemon.
- One teaspoon balsamic vinegar.
- 1/2 clove garlic, peeled and squashed.
- Few leaves basil, carefully chopped (or 1/2 teaspoon dried blended herbs to change basil and oregano).
- Few leaves oregano, carefully sliced.
- Generous flavoring of salt and freshly ground black pepper.

Directions:

1. Place the olives, garlic, purple potatoes, red onions, cucumbers, feta, peas, olives, yellow peppers, red ointment, cucumbers, and feta in each skewer.
2. Place all the dressing things needed in a little bowl and blend together thoroughly.
3. Put over the skewers.

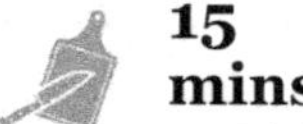 **15 mins**   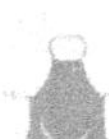 **20 mins**   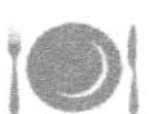 4   Calories: 220 - Fat: 3,8g - Fiber: 5g
Carbs: 38,9g - Protein: 7,1g

Chapter 14

Desserts

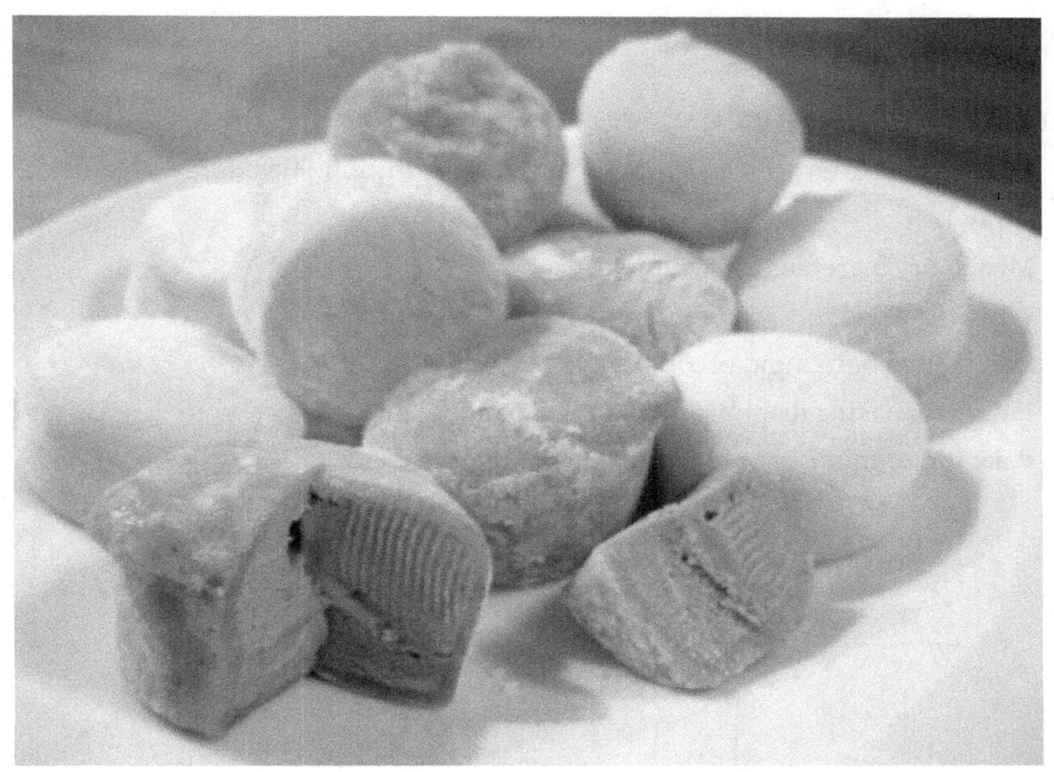

MATCHA MOCHI

Ingredients:

- 1 cup Superfine White Rice Flour
- 8 fl oz (250 ml) of coconut milk
- 2 tablespoons matcha powder
- 1/2 cup sugar
- 2 tablespoons butter melted
- 1 teaspoon baking powder

Directions:

1. Preheat the oven to 325.Spray baking dish with non-stick spray. (we use a coconut oil spray.).
2. Mix all dry ingredients, including sugar.
3. Whisk to blend.
4. Add melted butter and coconut milk. Stir well.
5. Put into a baking dish. We used an 8x8 pan.
6. Bake for 20 minutes or until done in the middle.

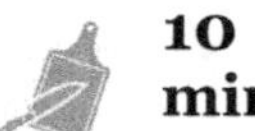 **10 mins**　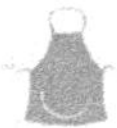 **20 mins**　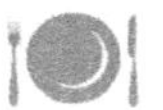 2　 Calories: 170 - Fat: 4,3g - Fiber: 3,9g
Carbs: 34g - Protein: 4,9g

CHOCO-MATCHA CUPCAKES

Ingredients:

- 5 ½ oz (150 g) coconut flour or almond flour
- 1/2 cup dates
- 2 oz (60 g) cocoa
- ½ tsp salt
- ½ tsp fine espresso coffee, decaf if preferred
- 4 fl oz (120 ml) milk
- ½ tsp vanilla extract
- 1 ½ fl oz (50 ml) vegetable oil
- 1 egg
- 4 fl oz (120 ml) boiling water
- 1 tsp baking powder

For the icing:

- 1 ½ oz (50 g) substitute sweetener
- 1 tbsp matcha green tea powder
- ½ tsp vanilla bean paste
- 1 ½ oz (50 g) chilled coconut cream, whipped

Directions:

1. Preheat the oven to 350° F/320° F fan. Line a cupcake tin with paper or silicone cake cases.
2. Place the flour, dates, cocoa, salt, and espresso powder in a large bowl and mix thoroughly.
3. Add the milk, vanilla extract, vegetable oil, and egg to the dry ingredients and use an electric mixer to beat until well combined.
4. Carefully pour in the boiling water slowly and beat on low speed until fully combined.
5. Use high speed to beat for a further minute to add air to the batter.
6. The batter is much more liquid than a normal cake mix.
7. Spoon the batter evenly between the cake cases. Each cake case should be no more than ¾ full. Bake in the oven for 15-18 minutes, until the mixture bounces back when tapped.
8. Remove from the oven and allow to cool completely before icing.
9. To make the icing, whip the coconut cream and icing sugar together until it's pale and smooth.
10. Add the matcha powder and vanilla and stir again. Pipe or spread over the cakes.

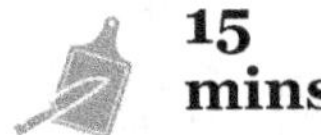 **15 mins**

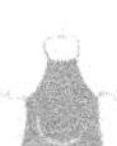 **15/18 mins**

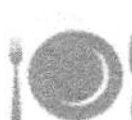 **12 pcs**

 Calories: 100 - Fat: 2,6g - Fiber: 1,4g
Carbs: 21,6g - Protein: 3,1g

Ingredients:

- 2½ cups whole walnuts
- ¼ cup almonds
- 2½ cups Medjoolodates

- 1 cup cacao powder
- 1 teaspoon vanilla extract
- ⅛-¼ teaspoon sea salt

Directions:

1. Place everything in a food processor until well combined.
2. Roll into balls and place on a baking sheet and freeze for 30 minutes or refrigerate for 2 hours.

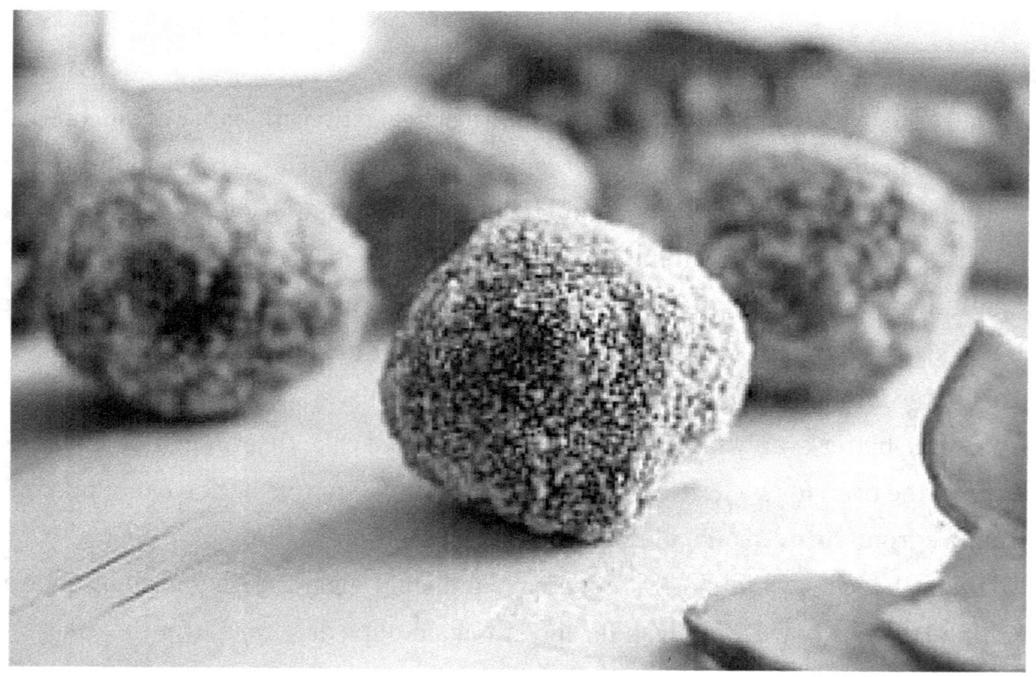

 **2 hrs.**  **0 mins** 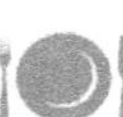 **12 pcs**  Calories: 110 - Fat: 2,8g - Fiber: 4,1g
Carbs: 31,6g - Protein: 5g

Ingredients:

- 9 oz (250 g) dark chocolate (85% cocoa solids)
- 6 medium free-range eggs, separated
- 4 tbsp strong black coffee
- 4 tbsp almond milk
- Chocolate coffee beans, to decorate

Directions:

1. Melt the chocolate in a large bowl set over a pan of gently simmering water, making sure the bottom of the bowl doesn't touch the water.
2. Remove the bowl from the heat and leave the melted chocolate to cool to room temperature. Once the melted chocolate is at room temperature, whisk in the egg yolks one at a time and then gently fold in the coffee and almond milk.
3. Using a hand-held electric mixer, whisk the egg whites until stiff peaks form, then mix a couple of tablespoons into the chocolate mixture to loosen it.
4. Gently fold in the remainder, using a large metal spoon.
5. Transfer the mousse to individual glasses and smooth the surface.
6. Cover with cling film and chill for at least 2 hours, ideally overnight.
7. Decorate with chocolate coffee beans before serving.

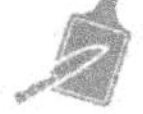 **2 hrs.** 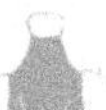 **15 mins** 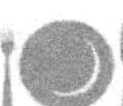 **12 pcs** 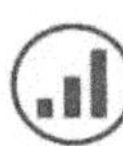 Calories: 156 - Fat: 3,1g - Fiber: 3,9g
Carbs: 3,1g - Protein: 3,6g

Ingredients:

- ½ cup almond flour
- ½ cup cooked quinoa
- 1/3 cup brown sugar
- ½ cup butter
- 4 tbsp tahini
- 16 dates, pitted and chopped
- 1 tsp baking soda
- ½ tsp vanilla extract

Directions:

1. Preheat oven to 350°F (180 C°).
2. Combine sugar, tahini, and butter stirring until creamy.
3. Add in remaining ingredients. Mix very well.
4. Spoon rounded teaspoonfuls of dough onto cookie sheets.
5. Bake for 10-12 minutes, or until cookies start to turn golden brown.

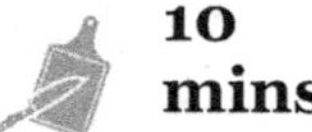 **10 mins** 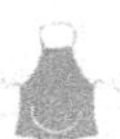 **10/12 mins** 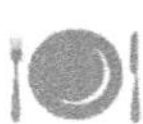 **12 pcs**  Calories: 176 - Fat: 1,5g - Fiber: 0,9g
Carbs: 27g - Protein: 1,5g

Ingredients:

- 4 oz (125 g) dark chocolate (min 85% cocoa)
- 11 oz (300 g) strawberries
- 7 oz (200 g) cherries
- 2 apples, peeled, cored and sliced
- 3½ fl oz (100 ml) double cream (heavy cream)

Directions:

1. Place the chocolate and cream into a fondue pot or saucepan and warm it until smooth and creamy.
2. Serve in the fondue pot or transfer it to a serving bowl.
3. Scatter the fruit on a serving dish ready to be dipped into the chocolate.

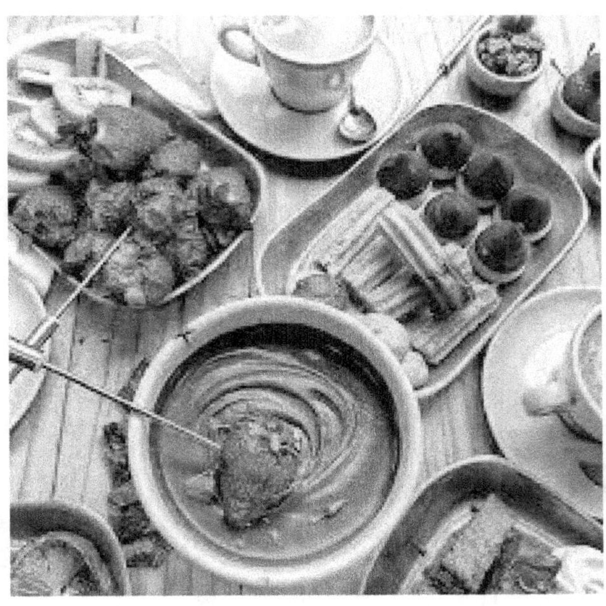

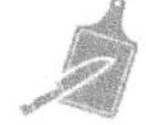 **10 mins** 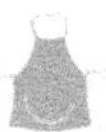 **10 mins** 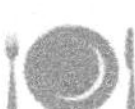 2 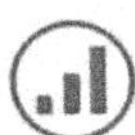 Calories: 129 - Fat: 3,1g - Fiber: 3,5g
Carbs: 28,5g - Protein: 3g

Ingredients:

- 250 g (9 oz) self-rising flour
- 125 g (4 oz) Medjool dates, chopped
- 50 g (2 oz) walnuts, chopped
- 250 ml (8 fl oz) milk
- 3 eggs
- 1 medium banana, mashed
- 1 tsp baking soda

Directions:

1. Sieve the baking soda and flour into a bowl.
2. Add in the banana, eggs, milk, and dates and combine all the ingredients thoroughly.
3. Transfer the mixture to a lined loaf tin and smooth it out.
4. Scatter the walnuts on top.
5. Bake the loaf in the oven at (180°C) 360°F for 45 minutes.
6. Transfer it to a wire rack to cool before serving.

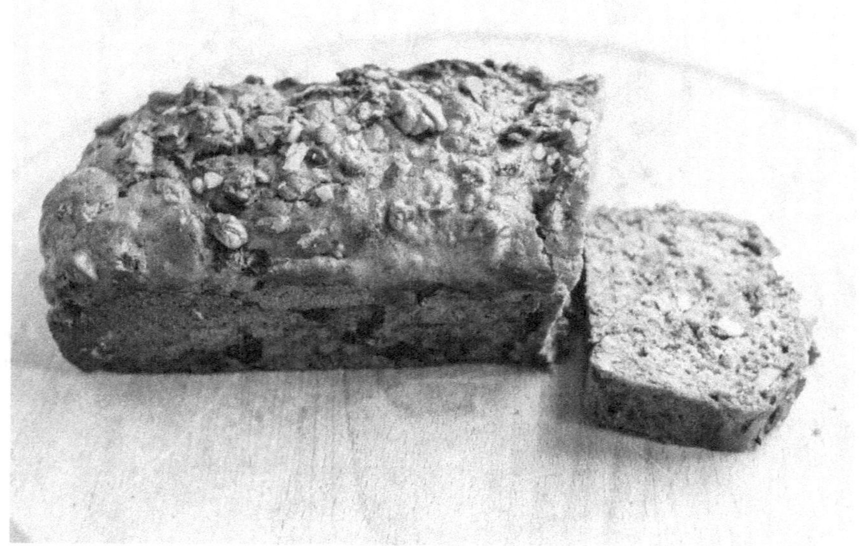

 **5 mins** 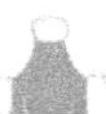 **45 mins** 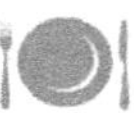 3

Calories: 178 - Fat: 4g - Fiber: 56g
Carbs: 45,8g - Protein: 3,5g

Ingredients:

- 2 apples
- 1 tbsp honey
- 2 star-anises
- 1 cinnamon sticks
- 5 fl oz (150 ml) green tea

Directions:

1. Place the honey and green tea into a saucepan and bring to the boil.
2. Add the apples, star anise, and cinnamon.
3. Reduce the heat and simmer gently for 15 minutes.
4. Serve the apples with a dollop of crème Fraiche or Greek yogurt.

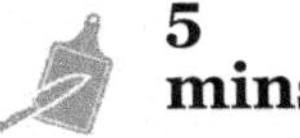 **5 mins** 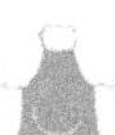 **5/10 mins** 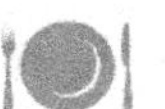 1 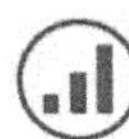 Calories: 120 - Fat: 1,7g - Fiber: 3,5g
Carbs: 28,5g - Protein: 3,8g

Ingredients:

- 2 medium firm apples, peeled and cut into ¼ inch slices
- 1 pie crust
- 1 ½ cups frozen berries (tayberries, raspberries, and blueberries)
- 4 teaspoons tapioca flour
- 1 teaspoon cinnamon
- 1/3 cup light brown sugar
- 1/3 cup white sugar
- ¼ teaspoon salt

Crumble Topping:

- ½ cup rolled oats
- 1/3 cup walnuts, chopped
- ½ cup all-purpose flour
- 6 tablespoons unsalted butter, cold and cut into cubes
- ¼ cup granulated sugar
- ¼ cup light brown sugar

Directions:

1. Preheat oven to 375° F (190° C). Line two 4-inch ceramic ramekins with rolled out pie crust.
2. Press crust into ramekins and repair any tears with extra pie crust.
3. Place in the freezer until ready to fill a pie. For Filling: Use a medium saucepan to combine apples and brown sugar.
4. Cook over medium-low heat for about 10 minutes, until reduced and bubbling.
5. Drain most juice from apples, and add berries, tapioca flour, sugar, cinnamon, and salt and stir gently to combine
6. For the crumble: Mix together all ingredients except butter.
7. Add butter and cut into the mixture with pastry cutter or fork until it resembles coarse crumbs.
8. Remove the pie crust from the freezer and add apple-berry filling until ramekin is full.
9. Add a generous handful of crumble topping by packing it on.
10. Bake for 25 minutes; the top of the pie should be starting to turn golden brown.
11. Tent with foil and bake for another 10 to 15 minutes until filling is bubbling.
12. Remove from the oven and let cool for 15 minutes. Serve warm and enjoy!

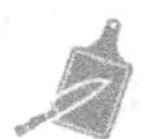 **20 mins** 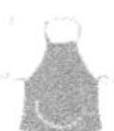 **1 hrs. & 15 mins** 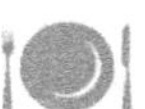 **2** Calories: 160 - Fat: 1,8g - Fiber: 4g
Carbs: 32g - Protein: 5g

STRAWBERRY COCONUT MOUSSE

Ingredients:

- 1 ¾ cups coconut cream
- 1 cup strawberries, diced
- 1-2 teaspoon granulated sweetener

Directions:

1. Whisk the coconut cream until fluffy and light.
2. In a small bowl, add the strawberries and sweetener.
3. Using the blade attachment on the stick blender, puree until smooth.
4. Gently fold the strawberry mixture with the fluffy coconut cream.
5. Serve in glasses and garnish with a few extra pieces of strawberry.
6. Refrigerate or freeze as you like.

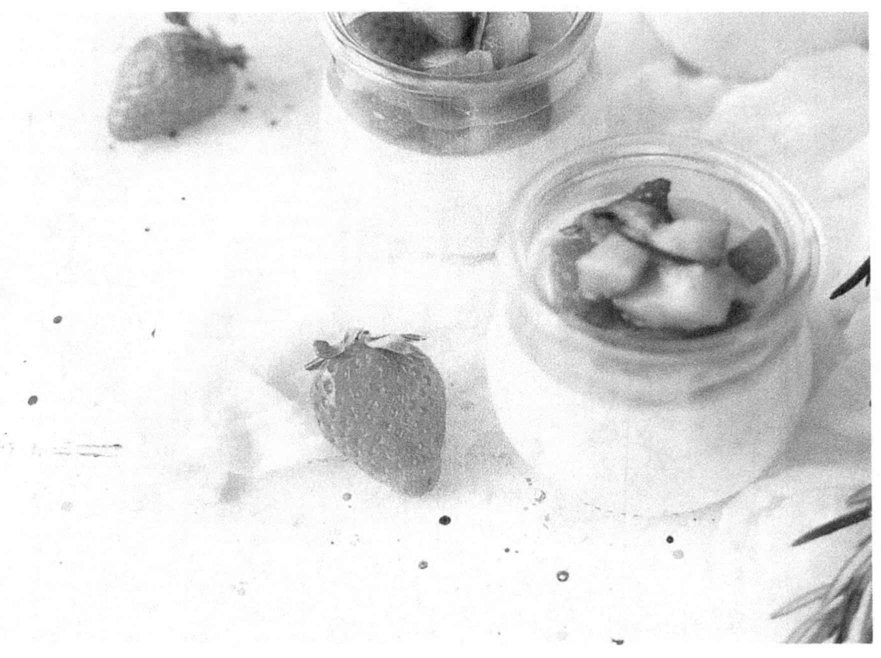

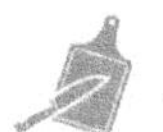 **15/20 mins**　　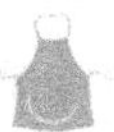 **0 mins**　　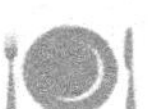 **4**　　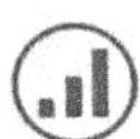　Calories: 145 - Fat: 3,5g - Fiber: 4,3g
Carbs: 34,8g - Protein: 4,8g

ESPRESSO GRANITA

Ingredients:

- 6 Espresso servings, at room temperature, short
- 3 Spoonfuls of sugar
- 3 cups ice
- 2 Cups hot water

Directions:

1. Pour espresso in a blender. Stir in the water.
2. Add the sugar and espresso together.
3. Stop the Mixer.
4. Add ice and water to taste.
5. Mix in until smooth.
6. Pour into cups to serve.
7. Willing to serve.

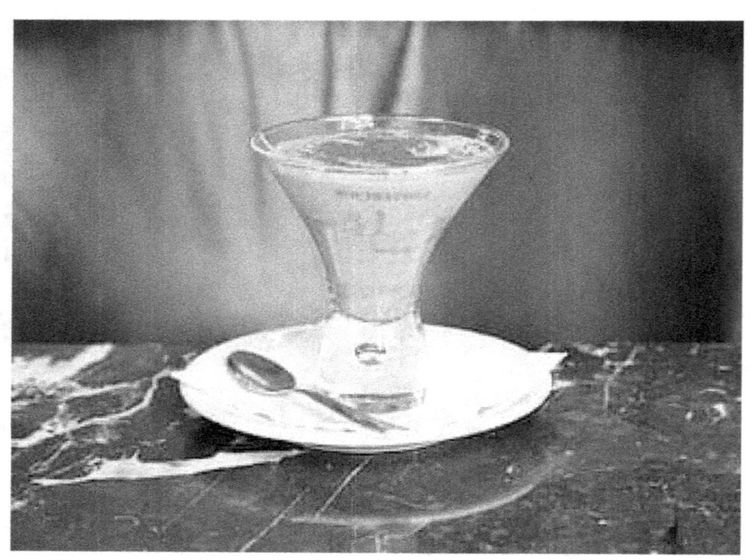

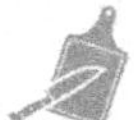 **15 mins**   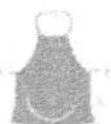 **0 mins**   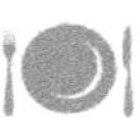 4   Calories: 90 - Fat: 0,5g - Fiber: 0,4g
Carbs: 21,5g - Protein: 0,1g

Ingredients:

- 2 fl oz (60 ml) Water
- 8 fl oz (250 ml) Coconut milk
- 3 tbsp Agar-agar
- 2 tbsp Raw honey or maple syrup
- 1 tsp Turmeric
- ½ tsp Ginger
- Pinch of cardamom powder
- Pinch of freshly ground black pepper

Directions:

1. Add the water to a big bowl and sprinkle the agar-agar on the water. Set the bowl aside.
2. Add the spices and the coconut milk to a saucepan placed over low-medium heat.
3. Whisk for about four to five minutes.
4. Put off the heat, then add the honey. Mix thoroughly.
5. Gently pour the milk mixture into the bowl that has the water and the agar-agar, then whisk until completely dissolved.
6. Transfer the mixture into a mold, preferably a pumpkin mold, then keep in the refrigerator for about three to four hours, until firm.
7. Place the gummies in an airtight container and keep in the fridge for up to one week.

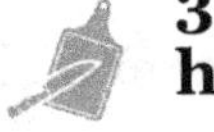 3/4 hrs.

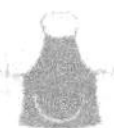 5 mins

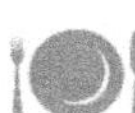 20 pcs

 Calories: 65 - Fat: 0,3g - Fiber: 0,1g
Carbs: 15g - Protein: 0,4g

Ingredients:

- 28 oz (800 g) Full-fat coconut milk cans
- 1 fl oz (30 ml) Extra virgin olive oil
- Maple syrup - 1/4 cup + more to taste
- Fresh ginger - 4 quarter-size slices
- A pinch of sea salt
- Ground cinnamon - ½ teaspoon
- Ground turmeric - 2 teaspoons
- Black pepper - 1/8 teaspoon
- Cardamom - 1/8 teaspoon (optional)
- Chopped candied ginger - 1/4 cup (optional)
- Pure vanilla extract - 1 teaspoon

Directions:

1. Place your ice cream churning bowl in the freezer a night before, to properly chill.
2. Add the maple syrup, turmeric, coconut milk, cardamom, fresh ginger, pepper, sea salt, and cinnamon into a large pot and heat over medium heat.
3. Allow simmering, whisking continuously to mix the ingredients. Then put off heat and add the vanilla extract. Stir once more to combine.
4. Adjust flavor if needed, adding more maple syrup for sweetness, turmeric for intense flavor, salt to balance the flavors, or cinnamon for warmth.
5. Transfer the mixture plus the ginger slices into a mixing bowl and allow to cool to room temperature.
6. Cover the bowl and place in the refrigerator to chill overnight or for a minimum of 4 to 6 hours.
7. The next day, use a strainer or a spoon to remove the ginger slices.
8. Then add the olive oil for more creaminess. Whisk to combine thoroughly.
9. Add the mixture to your ice cream maker and churn according to the instructions by the manufacturers – this should take about 30 minutes.
10. While the ice cream is churning, dice the candied ginger and add into the ice cream maker in the last few minutes of the churning.

11. Now move the ice cream to a big freezer-safe container and smoothen the top with your spoon.

12. Cover with a lid and place in the freezer for about four to six hours, until firm.

13. Bring out of the freezer ten minutes before serving to soften.

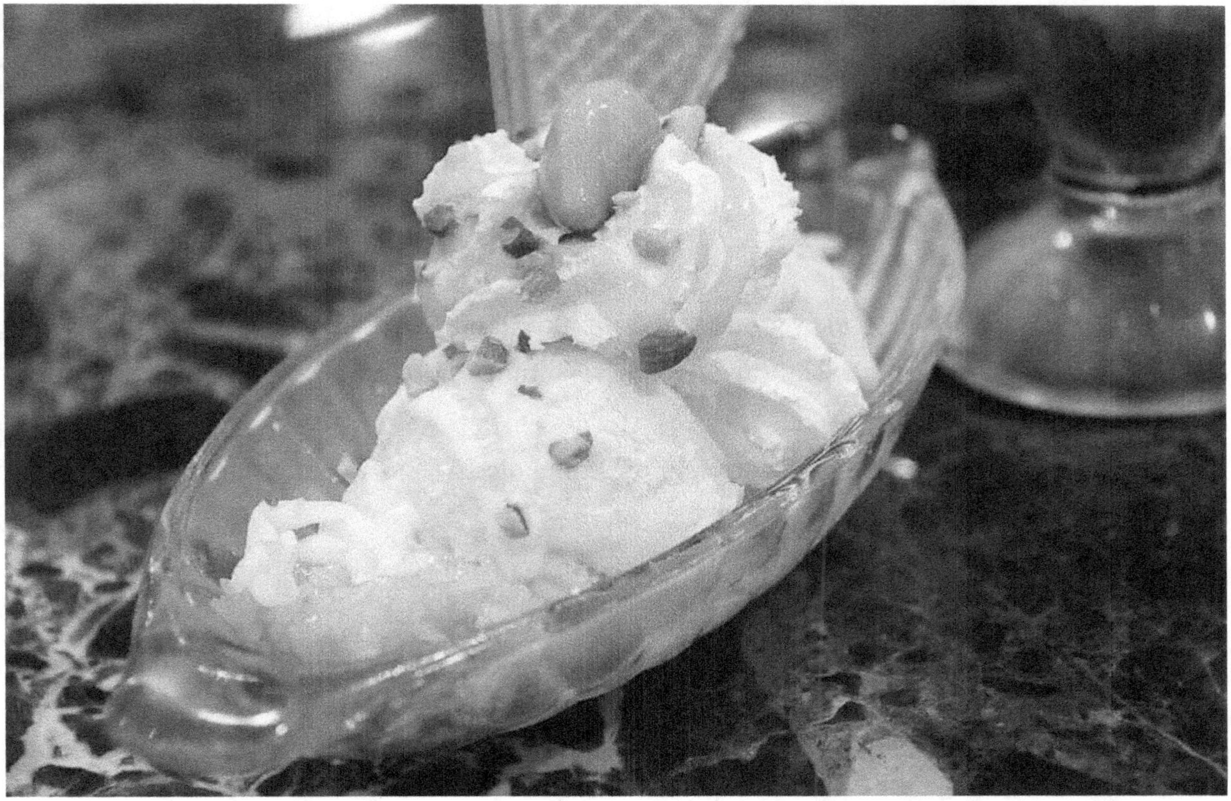

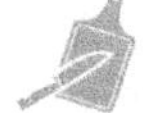

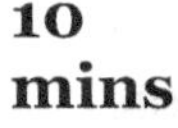 **10 mins**

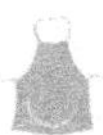 **8 hrs.**

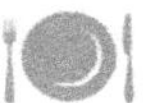 6

Calories: 100 - Fat: 3g - Fiber: 2g

Carbs: 29,1g - Protein: 2g

LEMON TOFU CHEESECAKE

Ingredients:

- 24 oz (680 ml) Silk tofu, drained
- 1 ½ tbsp Almond butter
- 1 cup Dates
- 1 tsp Lemon zest
- ½ tsp Sea salt
- ½ tsp Vanilla extract
- 1 fl oz (30 ml) Lemon juice
- 1 ½ tbsp Cornstarch
- 1 pc Crust, 8-inch

Directions:

1. Preheat the oven to Fahrenheit three-hundred and fifty degrees. If you are preparing the lemon tofu cheesecake without a crust, I recommend preparing eight individual ramekins to divide the filling between.

2. Otherwise, make an eight-inch crust of your choice. Whisk together the lemon juice with the cornstarch to form a slurry.

3. In a food processor or blender, combine the cornstarch slurry and remaining ingredients until fully combined, smooth, and creamy. You don't want any lumps.

4. Pour the lemon tofu cheesecake filling into the prepared crust or ramekins if baking with the crust allows the cheesecake to cook until set, about thirty minutes.

5. On the other hand, if you are using individual ramekins, the cheesecake will only take fifteen to twenty- two minutes, depending on the size of the ramekins.

6. Allow the cheesecake to cool to room temperature, and then transfer it to the fridge until completely chilled through.

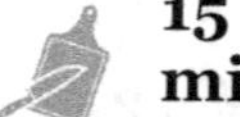 **15 mins**

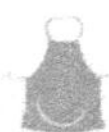 **15/30 mins**

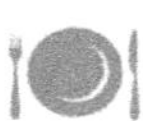 **8**

Calories: 240 - Fat: 4g - Fiber: 7g
Carbs: 43g - Protein: 3g

BLUEBERRY WALNUT CRISP

Ingredients:

- ¼ cup Walnuts, chopped
- ½ cup Rolled oats
- 2 tbsp Date sugar
- ½ tsp cinnamon, ground
- ¼ tsp Sea salt
- 2 tbsp butter, cut into cubes

- 4 cups Blueberries
- 1 tbsp Cornstarch
- 2 tbsp Date sugar
- ½ tsp Lemon zest
- 1 tsp Vanilla extract

Directions:

1. Begin by preheating your oven to 350° F (190 C°) and preparing six individual ramekins with non-stick cooking spray. Set the ramekins on a baking sheet to avoid spilling.
2. In a bowl, toss together the blueberries with the cornstarch, date sugar, lemon zest, and vanilla.
3. Once combined, divide the blueberries between the ramekins.
4. To make the crispy topping combine the remaining ingredients with a fork or pastry cutter. It will be crumbly.
5. Top the blueberries in the ramekins with the crumble.
6. Set the baking sheet of ramekins in the oven and bake until golden- brown, about twenty-five to thirty minutes.
7. Remove the blueberry walnut crisp from the oven and allow the crisps to cool slightly before serving.

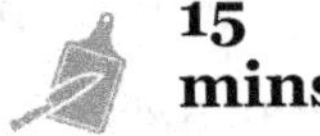 15 mins

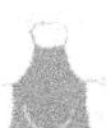 35 mins

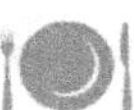 6

Calories: 175 - Fat: 3g - Fiber: 3,1g
Carbs: 34,6g - Protein: 3,8g

Ingredients:

- 2 cups of oats/flakes that are ready without cooking
- 1 cup of blackcurrants without the stems
- 1 tsp of honey (or ¼ tsp of raw sugar)
- 4 fl oz (120 ml) of water (add more or less by testing the pan)
- 1 cup of plain yogurt (or soy or coconut)

Directions:

1. Boil the berries, honey, and water and then turn it down on low.
2. Put in a glass container in a refrigerator until it is cool and set (about 30 minutes or more)
3. When ready to eat, scoop the berries on top of the oats and yogurt.
4. Serve immediately.

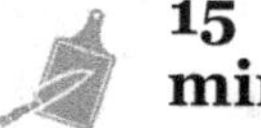 **15 mins** 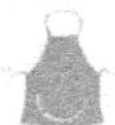 **35 mins** 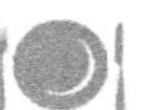 6  Calories: 160 - Fat: 2,7g - Fiber: 4,1g
Carbs: 30g - Protein: 5,4g

Chapter 15

Snacks

HONEY CHILI NUTS

Ingredients:

- 5 oz (150 g) walnuts
- 5 oz (150 g) pecan nuts
- 2 oz (50 g) softened butter
- 1 tablespoon honey
- ½ bird's-eye chili, very finely chopped and deseeded

Directions:

1. Preheat the oven to (180° C) 360° F.
2. Combine the butter, honey, and chili in a bowl, then add the nuts and stir them well.
3. Spread the nuts onto a lined baking sheet and roast them in the oven for 10 minutes, stirring once halfway through.
4. Remove from the oven and allow them to cool before eating.

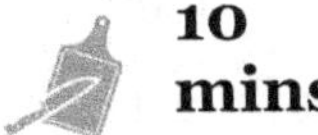 **10 mins** 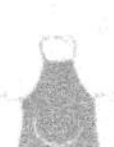 **30 mins** 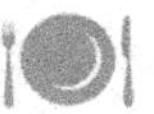 4 Calories: 126 - Fat: 0,5g - Fiber: 0,8g
Carbs: 4,9g - Protein: 2g

Ingredients:

- 1 – 6.5 oz jar artichoke hearts, drained and chopped
- ½ cup pizza sauce, preferably with garlic
- 2 tablespoons fresh cilantro
- ¾ cup Parmesan cheese, grated
- 1/3 cup light mayonnaise

Directions:

1. Heat oven to 350° F (180 C°).
2. Mix all of the dip ingredients together and spoon into a shallow ovenproof dish or 9-inch pie plate sprayed with non-stick cooking spray.
3. Bake 20 minutes until hot and bubbly.
4. Garnish with cilantro sprigs and serve warm.
5. Serve with chips, nachos, bread, or veggies. Enjoy!

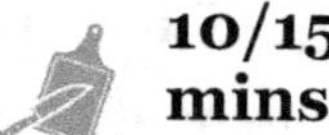 **10/15 mins** 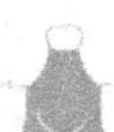 **20 mins** 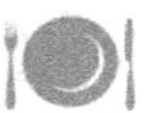 6  Calories: 81 - Fat: 5,4g - Fiber: 1,6g
Carbs: 34g - Protein: 2,1g

Ingredients:

- 2 tbsp (1 fl oz – 30 ml) extra virgin olive oil
- ½ teaspoon onion powder
- ½ teaspoon turmeric
- ½ teaspoon ground cumin
- 1 medium head cauliflower
- ¾ cup shredded cheddar cheese
- ½ cup tomato, diced
- ¼ cup red bell pepper, diced
- ¼ cup red onion, diced
- ½ Bird's Eye chili pepper, finely diced
- ¼ cup parsley, finely diced
- Pinch of salt

Directions:

1. Preheat oven to 400 ° F (200 ° C).
2. Mix onion powder, cumin, turmeric, and olive oil.
3. Core cauliflower and slice into ½" thick rounds.
4. Coat the cauliflower with the olive oil mixture and bake for 15 – 20 minutes.
5. Top with shredded cheese & bake for an additional 3 – 5 minutes, until cheese is melted.
6. In a bowl, combine tomatoes, bell pepper, onion, chili, and parsley with a pinch of salt.
7. Top cooked cauliflower with salsa and serve.

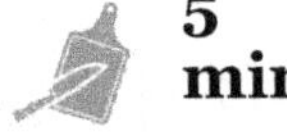 5 mins

 30 mins

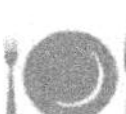 1/2

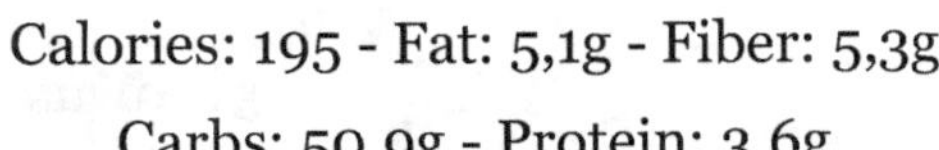
Calories: 195 - Fat: 5,1g - Fiber: 5,3g
Carbs: 50,9g - Protein: 3,6g

Ingredients:

- 2 cups rolled oats
- ½ cup raisins
- ½ cup walnuts, chopped and toasted
- 1 ½ teaspoon ground cardamom
- 6 tablespoons cocoa butter
- 1/3 cup packed brown sugar
- 3 tablespoons honey
- Coconut oil, for greasing pan

Directions:

1. Preheat oven to 350° F (180 C°).
2. Line a 9-inch square pan with foil, extending the foil over the sides.
3. Grease the foil with coconut oil. Mix the oats, raisins, walnuts, and cardamom in a large bowl.
4. Heat the cocoa butter, brown sugar, and honey in a saucepan until the butter melts and begins to bubble.
5. Bake for 30 minutes or until the top is golden brown.
6. Allow cooling for 30 minutes.
7. Using the foil, lift the granola out of the pan and place on cutting board.
8. Cut into 18 bars.

 **5 mins** 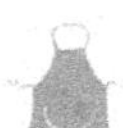 **30 mins** 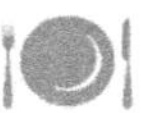 **18 pcs** 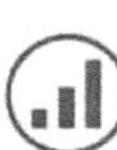 Calories: 95 - Fat: 2g - Fiber: 1,8g
Carbs: 7,8g - Protein: 3g

Ingredients:

- ½ cauliflower head, riced
- 1/3 cup low-fat mozzarella cheese, shredded
- ¼ cup egg whites
- 1 teaspoon Italian dressing, low fat
- Pepper to taste

Directions:

1. Spread cauliflower rice over a lined baking sheet.
2. Preheat your oven to 375° F (190° C). Roast for 20 minutes.
3. Transfer to a bowl and spread pepper, cheese, seasoning, egg whites, and stir well.
4. Spread in a rectangular pan and press.
5. Transfer to oven and cook for 20 minutes more. Serve and enjoy!

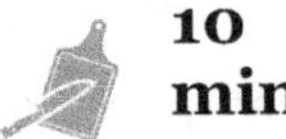 **10 mins** 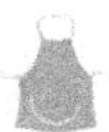 **40 mins** 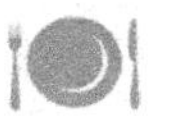 1  Calories: 90 - Fat: 4g - Fiber: 1,7g
Carbs: 3,8g - Protein: 4g

Ingredients:

- 90 oz (250 g) kale, chopped into approx. 2 in (4 cm)
- 2 oz (50 g) ground almonds
- 2 oz (50 g) parmesan cheese
- 3 tbsp tomato purée (tomato paste)
- ½ tsp mixed herbs
- ½ tsp oregano
- ½ tsp onion powder
- 2 tbsp olive oil
- 3 ½ fl oz (100 ml) water

Directions:

1. Place all of the ingredients, except the kale, into the food processor and process until finely chopped into a smooth consistency.
2. Toss the kale leaves in the parmesan mixture, coating it really well.
3. Spread the kale out onto 2 baking sheets.
4. Bake in the oven at (170 °C) 325° F for 15 minutes, until crispy.

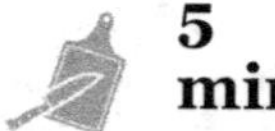 **5 mins** 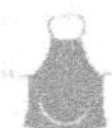 **15 mins** 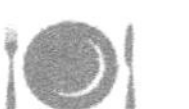 1 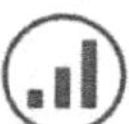 Calories: 78 - Fat: 7,1g - Fiber: 1,3g
Carbs: 4g - Protein: 3,1g

Ingredients:

- ½ cup walnuts
- ½ cup coconut flakes
- ½ tsp soy sauce
- 1 tsp honey
- 1 pinch of cayenne pepper
- 1 dash of lime juice

Directions:

1. Add the above ingredients to a bowl, toss the nuts to coat, and place on a baking sheet, lined with parchment paper.
2. Cook at 250° F (120° C) for 15-20 minutes, checking as not to burn, but lightly toasted.
3. Remove from the oven.
4. Cool first before eating.

 **5 mins** 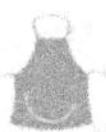 **15/20 mins**  2 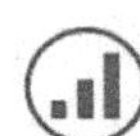

Calories: 56 - Fat: 0,5g - Fiber: 0,8g
Carbs: 5,1g - Protein: 4g

DATE & WALNUT CINNAMON BITES

Ingredients:

- 3 walnut halves
- 3 pitted Medjool dates
- the ground cinnamon, to taste

Directions:

1. Cut each walnut carefully into three slices, and do the same with dates.
2. Put a slice of walnut, brush with cinnamon, and serve.

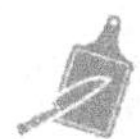 **5 mins** 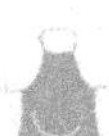 **0 mins** 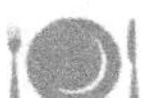 1 

Calories: 78 - Fat: 7g - Fiber: 0,9g
Carbs: 3,4g - Protein: 1,5g

Ingredients:

- 7 oz (200 g) whole oats.
- 1 ½ oz (50 g) pecans, approximately. Sliced
- 3 tbsp (1 ½ fl oz – 50 ml) light olive oil.

- ¾ oz (20 g) butter.
- 1 tablespoon dark brown sugar.
- 2 tablespoon rice malt syrup.
- 2 oz (60 g) good-quality (70%), Dark chocolate chips.

Directions:

1. The oven is preheated to 320° F (300° F fan/gas 3).
2. Cover a large bakery with a silicone surface or pastry.
3. The olive oil, butter, brown sugar, and rice malt syrup should be gently heated in a little non-adhesive pot until the butter has finally cooled, and sugar and syrup have properly dissolved.
4. Pour the syrup over the oats and stir until the oats are completely covered.
5. Distribute the granola over the bakery and extend it into the corners. Leave mixed clumps of overlapping instead of even scattering.
6. Bake in the microwave for 20 minutes till just tinged golden brown at the edges.
7. Get rid of the microwave oven and leave to cool on the tray entirely.
8. When cool, break up any bigger swellings on the tray with your fingers and, after that, blend in the chocolate chips.
9. Scoop or put the granola into an airtight tub or jar.
10. The granola will keep for a minimum of 2 weeks.

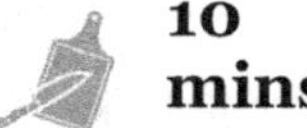 **10 mins** 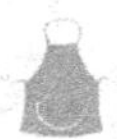 **30 mins**  **3/4**  Calories: 90 - Fat: 6,5g - Fiber: 1,4g
Carbs: 3,4g - Protein: 3g

Ingredients:

- 1 cup old fashion ginger, dried (I've used apple cinnamon-flavored oats also)
- 1/4 cup quinoa cooked using 3/4 cup orange juice
- 1 Tbsp reduced-fat peanut butter
- 1/4 cup shredded unsweetened coconut
- 1/3 cup dried cranberry/raisin blend
- 1/3 cup dark chocolate chips
- 1/4 cup slivered almonds

Directions:

1. Cook quinoa in orange juice.
2. Bring to boil and simmer for approximately 1-2 minutes. Let cool.
3. Combine chilled quinoa and the remaining ingredients into a bowl.
4. With wet hands and combine ingredients and roll in golden ball sized chunks.
5. Set at a Tupperware and set in the refrigerator for two weeks until the firm.

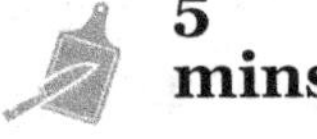 5 mins 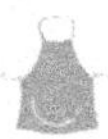 5 mins  2/4 

Calories: 80 - Fat: 7g - Fiber: 1g
Carbs: 3,5g - Protein: 2,5g

Ingredients:

- 1 tsp vanilla extract or the scraped seeds of 1 vanilla pod
- 1 tbsp (1/2 oz – 15 ml) of extra virgin olive oil
- 1 tbsp of ground turmeric
- 1 tbsp of cocoa powder

- 9 oz (250 g) of pitted Medjool dates
- 1 oz (30 g) of dark chocolate or cocoa nibs (85% cocoa solids), broken into pieces
- 4 ½ oz (120 g) of walnuts
- 1–2 tbsp (1/2 – 1 fl oz) of water

Directions:

1. Pulse the chocolate and walnuts in a food processor until the texture resembles a fine powder.
2. Add the vanilla extract, ground turmeric, cocoa powder, olive oil, and Medjool dates and pulse until a ball is formed.
3. Add water if the consistency is sticky.
4. Mold the mixture with your hands into bite-sized balls, transfer into an airtight container and refrigerate for at least 60 minutes before consuming. If desired, coat balls in cocoa or desiccated coconut. You can store it in your fridge for up to 1 week.

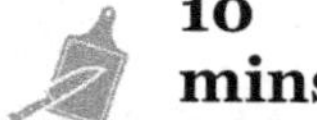 **10 mins** 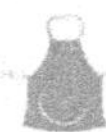 **65 mins** 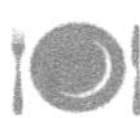 **20 pcs**  Calories: 76 - Fat: 6,8g - Fiber: 0,9g
Carbs: 2,7g - Protein: 2,3g

Ingredients:

- 2 x 14 oz cans (400 g each) of butter beans, drained and rinsed
- 3 tbsp (1 ½ fl oz – 50 ml) extra virgin olive oil
- 2 tablespoons brown miso paste
- juice and grated zest of 1/2 unwaxed lemon
- 4 medium scallions, trimmed and finely chopped
- 1 garlic clove, crushed
- 1/4 Thai chili, finely chopped celery sticks, to serve
- oatcakes, to serve

Directions:

1. Simply mash the first seven ingredients together with a potato masher until you have a coarse mixture.
2. Serve as a dip with celery sticks and oatcakes.

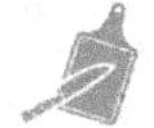 **15 mins** 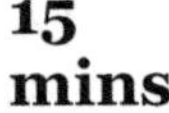 **0 mins** 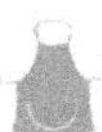 **4** 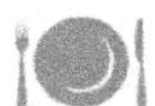  Calories: 110 - Fat: 7,3g - Fiber: 2,1g
Carbs: 8g - Protein: 3,9g

Ingredients:

- 5 oz (100 g) kale, stalks taken off, thoroughly washed and dried
- 1 tsp dried garlic granules
- 1/2 tsp salt
- 1 tbsp (1/2 oz – 15 ml) olive oil
- 1/2 tsp chili flakes (optional, leave out if you don't like them spicy)
- 1 tbsp nutritional yeast flakes (optional)

Directions:

1. Preheat the oven to (150° C) 300° F.
2. Thoroughly wash and dry the kale, as if it is left damp, it will not crisp up as much when baking.
3. Remove any woody stalks and break into bite-sized pieces approx. 2 inches or whatever you prefer.
4. Place the prepared kale in a bowl and drizzle over the olive and sprinkle over the remaining ingredients.
5. Now massage the ingredients in, making sure the leaves are thoroughly coated.
6. Lay the coated kale onto two baking trays, making sure the leaves don't overlap, as a bit of space allows the chips to crisp up best.
7. Cook for 7 minutes, then rotate the tray and cook for a further 7 minutes.
8. Allow to cool slightly and enjoy.

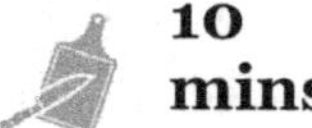 **10 mins** 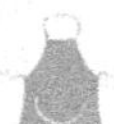 15 mins 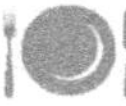 2/4  Calories: 70 - Fat: 4,9g - Fiber: 1,4g
Carbs: 5,3g - Protein: 2,6g

Basic Snacks for Sirt Boost

Red grapes	10 pcs (30 calories)
Apple	1 pc (47 calories)
Green Tea	1 cup (0 calories)
Cocoa	2 tsp (33 calories)
5 Olives	Six large black or green olives (75 calories)
Blackberries	15 blackberries (32 cals)
Blueberries	25 blueberries (36 cals)
Pomegranate seeds	50g/half a small pack (50 calories)
Dark chocolate 85%	Six squares/20g chocolate (125 calories)

Chapter 16

Dressings and Sauces

"SIRTIFIED" MUSTARD

Ingredients:

- ¼ cup Apple cider vinegar
- 1 tbsp raw honey
- ½ cup Ground mustard
- ¼ tsp Ground turmeric

Directions:

1. Stir all ingredients until well combined in a small mixing bowl.
2. May be kept in a well-sealed jar in the fridge.

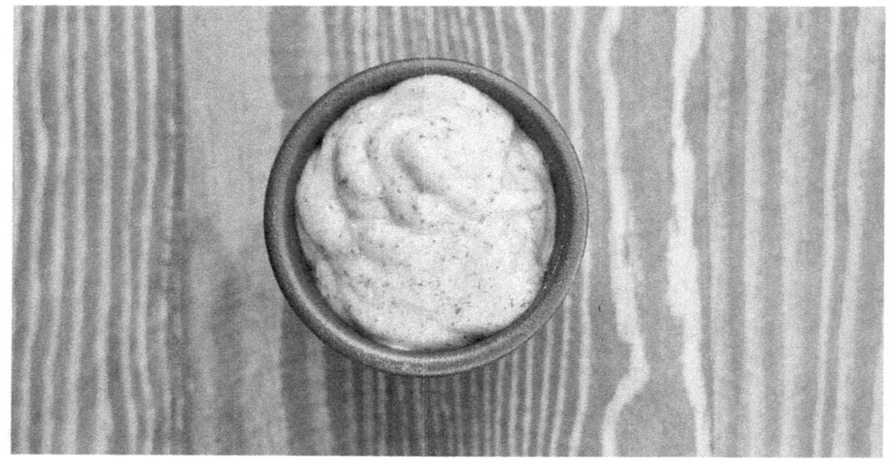

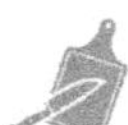 **5/10 mins**  **0 mins** 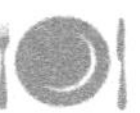 1 Calories: 50 - Fat: 1,3g - Fiber: 0,6g
Carbs: 9g - Protein: 2g

Ingredients:

- 1 can Coconut cream
- 2 tbsp Shallots minced
- 1/8 cup Chives chopped
- 2 ½ tbsp (1 ¼ fl oz – 40 ml) Apple cider vinegar

- 1 ½ tbsp basil, chopped
- 3 tsp Dill, chopped
- 2 tbsp Parsley chopped
- ¼ tsp Fine sea salt
- 1 clove Garlic, minced

Directions:

1. Open the coconut cream and scoop out the cream leaving the water in the can.
2. Whisk together the cream with the 4 Tablespoons of the coconut water.
3. Once well combined, mix the remaining items on the list of ingredients into the bowl and blend together until they are well blended. Before serving, allow the flavors to combine by storing in the fridge for at least 30 minutes.

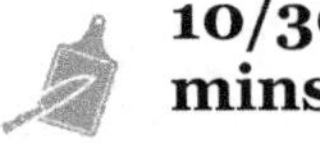 **10/30 mins**

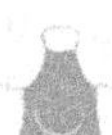 **0 mins**

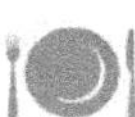 **4/5**

Calories: 43 - Fat: 0,5g - Fiber: 1g
Carbs: 6,8g - Protein: 3g

Ingredients:

- 1/3 cup (2 ½ fl oz – 80 ml) Olive oil
- ¼ cup (2 fl oz – 60 ml) Water
- ¼ cup (2 fl oz – 60 ml) Apple cider vinegar
- 1 tsp Dried basil
- ½ cup Raspberries
- 1 tsp Fine sea salt

Directions:

1. Combine all items from the list of ingredients in a blender and mix together until they reach a smooth consistency.

 **5 mins** 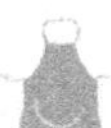 **0 mins**  **2** 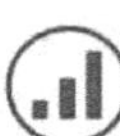 Calories: 39 - Fat: 0,37g - Fiber: 0,8g
Carbs: 8g - Protein: 3g

Ingredients:

- 2 tbsp (1 oz – 30 ml) Lemon juice
- 1/3 cup (2 ½ fl oz – 80 ml) Extra virgin olive oil
- 1 tsp ground turmeric
- 2 tsp raw honey
- ½ cup Avocado
- ¼ tsp Sea salt

Directions:

1. Combine all ingredients together in a blender.
2. The avocado will make it a thicker dressing or dip.
3. Add in until it reaches your desired consistency.

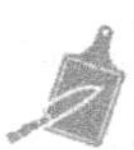 **5 mins** 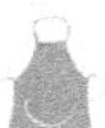 **0 mins**  **2**  Calories: 45,8 - Fat: 0,6g - Fiber: 1g
Carbs: 10g - Protein: 5g

Ingredients:

- 12 oz (350 g) Carrot
- 6 oz (170 g) Beets
- 2 tbsp Honey
- ¼ cup (2 fl oz – 60 ml) No sugar added apple juice
- ½ tsp Sea salt

- 1 ¼ tbsp (1/3 fl oz – 20 ml) Apple cider vinegar
- ½ tsp Powdered onion
- ¼ tsp Powdered ginger
- ¼ tsp Powdered garlic

Directions:

1. Insert a steaming basket over a large pot and add water to just about an inch below the steamer.
2. Put the beets and carrots in the basket and heat water to boiling.
3. Once boiling, turn down the burner to low/midlevel and allow to cook for 12-15 additional minutes covered.
4. Once the vegetables are soft, remove them from the steamer and combine them in a blender with the remaining items on the list of the ingredients.
5. Pulse and mix until you get a smooth sauce.
6. Pour the "ketchup" into a small saucepan, cook on a low simmer for 18-20 minutes at medium-low heat. "Ketchup" may be kept in a well-sealed glass jar no longer than 3 days in the refrigerator. Or store in the freezer and thaw out as needed.

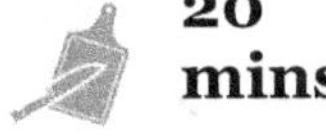 **20 mins**  **40 mins** 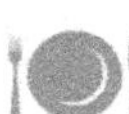 2/4　Calories: 45,9 - Fat: 0,6g - Fiber: 0,5g
Carbs: 8,9g - Protein: 4g

Ingredients:

- ½ cup (4 fl oz – 120 ml) Water
- ½ cup Cashews, raw
- 2 cups Cilantro, chopped
- 1 pc Jalapeno, chopped
- 7 oz (200 g) Green chilies, canned
- 1 ½ tsp (2/3 fl oz – 25 ml) Apple cider vinegar
- 1 tsp Sea salt

Directions:

1. Soak the cashews.
2. To do this, either cover them with water and allow them to sit covered for six to twelve hours, or simmer them on the stove in water for fifteen minutes.
3. Drain off the water and add the cashews to a blender.
4. Into the blender, add the remaining ingredients, and blend the enchilada sauce until it is completely smooth.
5. Use the green enchilada sauce immediately or store it in the refrigerator for up to a week.

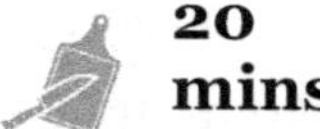 **20 mins**   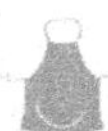 **15 mins**   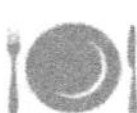 **5/6**   Calories: 38,6 - Fat: 1g - Fiber: 0,9g
Carbs: 7g - Protein: 1,4g

Ingredients:

- 2 tablespoons minced shallots
- 2 teaspoons fine ocean salt
- 1/4 teaspoon newly ground dark pepper
- 1 cup pecans, daintily toasted (see Note underneath)
- 1 cup (8 fl oz – 250 ml) of water
- 1/2 cup (4 fl oz – 120 ml) sherry vinegar
- 1/2 cup (4 fl oz – 120 ml) imported pecan oil
- 1/2 cup (4 fl oz – 120 ml) vegetable oil

Directions:

1. Put all ingredients in a blender, except for the oil and blitz at high speed.
2. With the machine running, slowly put in the olive and pecan oils until the vinaigrette is emulsified.
3. Refrigerate to prepare for serving.

 **5 mins** 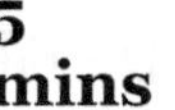 **0 mins**  **4/6** 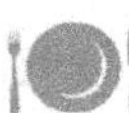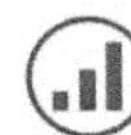 Calories: 35 - Fat: 0,5g - Fiber: 0,8g
Carbs: 6,5g - Protein: 1,9g

Ingredients:

- 2 tsp ground turmeric
- 1 tsp ground ginger
- 5 tbsp (2 ½ fl oz – 75 ml) Avocado Oil
- ½ tsp garlic powder
- Juice of three little lemons (simply over ¼ c of a replacement squeeze)
- 1 tbsp Honey
- Salt to taste

Directions:

1. Place all ingredients in a blender.
2. At that time, mix well. Don't hesitate to vary your seasonings as per need.
3. Pour over the flame-broiled vegetables, greens keep the extra dressing in the chiller.

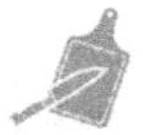 **5 mins** 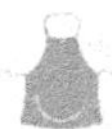 **0 mins** 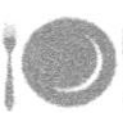 **2/4** 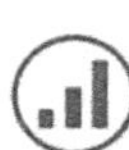 Calories: 41 - Fat: 0,7g - Fiber: 0,3g
Carbs: 5,1g - Protein: 3g

Ingredients:

- 3/4 cup plain yogurt
- 2 tbsp. chopped fresh cilantro
- 3/4 tsp. ground coriander
- 1 chopped scallion
- 3/4 tsp. cumin
- 1/2 seeded, coarsely grated, and peeled English cucumber
- Kosher salt and black pepper

Directions:

1. Place all ingredients in a blender.
2. At that time, mix well. Don't hesitate to vary your seasonings as per need.
3. Add in the salt and black pepper.
4. Now serve and enjoy.

 **10 mins**  **0 mins**  **3/4** 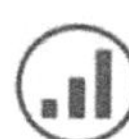 Calories: 57 - Fat: 0,3g - Fiber: 0,2g
Carbs: 15g - Protein: 0,4g

Ingredients:

- 1/3 cup avocado, mashed
- 2 cloves garlic, minced
- 1 tbsp (1/2 fl oz – 15 ml) olive oil
- 2 anchovy fillets or 1 teaspoon anchovy paste
- 3 tbsp (1 ½ fl oz – 45 ml) lemon juice
- ¼ cup Parmesan cheese, shredded or shaved
- ½ teaspoon mustard
- 2 tablespoons unsweetened almond milk
- 2 tsp (1/3 fl oz) Worcestershire sauce
- 2 tbsp (1 fl oz – 30 ml) water
- ¾ teaspoon sea salt
- ¼ teaspoon ground pepper

Directions:

1. Add all ingredients into a high-powered blender or food processor and blend until smooth.
2. Taste and add additional salt and pepper if needed.

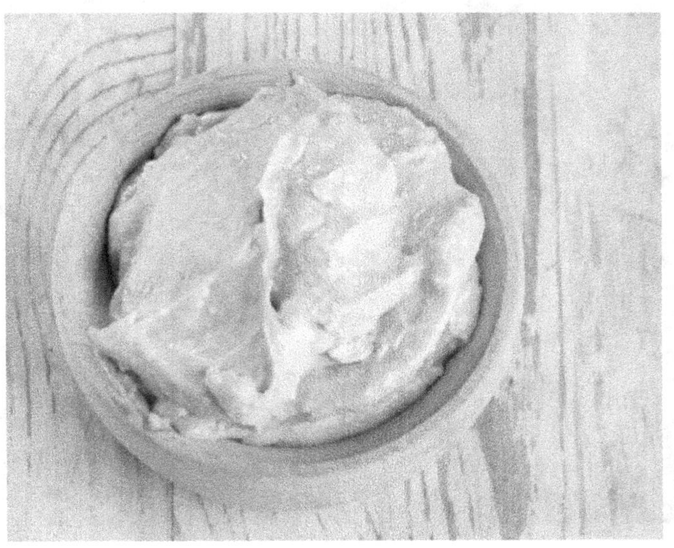

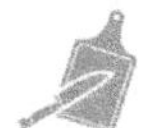 **10 mins** 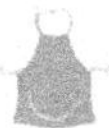 **0 mins** 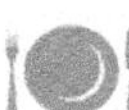 **3/4**  Calories: 58 - Fat: 2g - Fiber: 1,5g
Carbs: 8g - Protein: 1g

Ingredients:

- 8 oz (230 g) cream cheese
- 2 teaspoons (1/3 fl oz – 10 ml) olive oil
- ½ lemon, the zest
- 1 clove garlic
- ½ cup fresh parsley or fresh basil, chopped
- Salt and pepper to taste

Directions:

1. Stir all ingredients into the cream cheese.
2. Let sit in the refrigerator for at least 10 minutes to let all the flavors develop.
3. Add salt if needed.

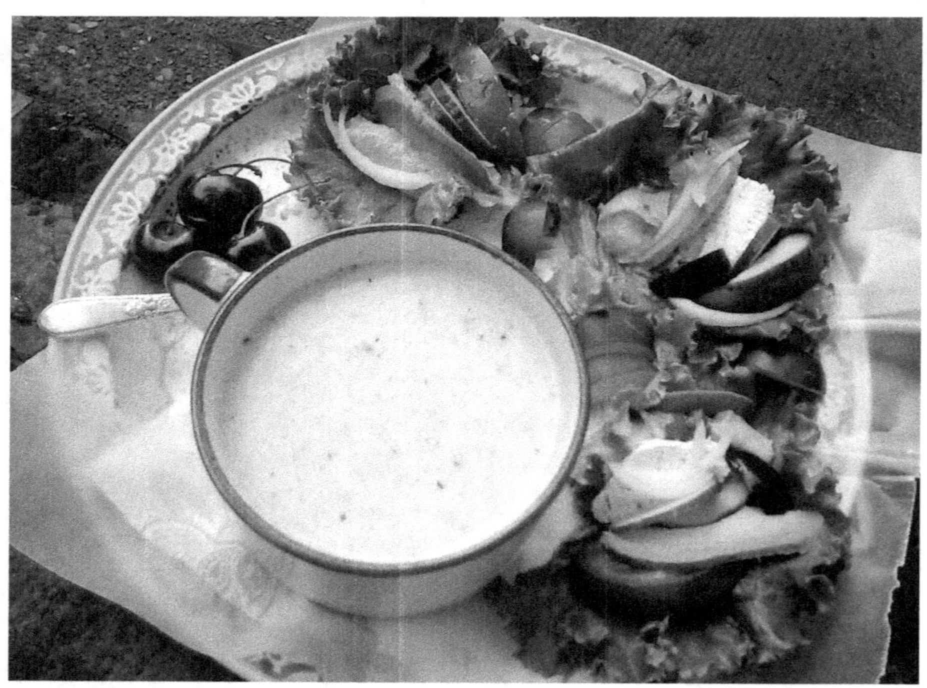

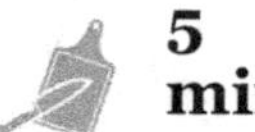 **5 mins**   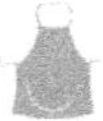 **0 mins**   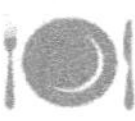 **4**   Calories: 41 - Fat: 0,7g - Fiber: 0,3g
Carbs: 5,1g - Protein: 3g

Ingredients:

- 1 ½ cups creamy peanut butter
- 3 cloves garlic, minced
- ½ cup (4 fl oz – 120 ml) of coconut milk
- 3 tbsp (1 ½ fl oz – 50 ml) fresh lime juice
- ¼ cup fresh cilantro, chopped
- 1 tablespoon fresh ginger root, minced
- 1 tbsp (1/2 fl oz – 15 ml) hot sauce
- 3 tbsp (1 ½ fl oz – 50 ml) water
- 1 tbsp (1/2 fl oz – 15 ml) fish sauce

Directions:

1. In a bowl, mix the peanut butter, coconut milk, water, lime juice, soy sauce, fish sauce, hot sauce, ginger, and garlic.
2. Mix in the cilantro just before serving.

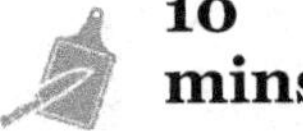 **10 mins**  **0 mins** 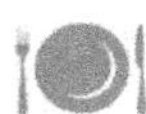 **8/10** 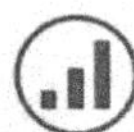 Calories: 57 - Fat: 2,4g - Fiber: 1,6g
Carbs: 19,5g - Protein: 2g

Ingredients:

- 1 cup avocado mayonnaise
- 1 tablespoon Italian seasoning

Italian Seasoning

- 3 tablespoons dried oregano
- 3 tablespoons dried parsley
- 3 tablespoons dried basil
- 1 tablespoon garlic powder

- 1 teaspoon dried thyme
- 1 teaspoon dried rosemary
- 1 teaspoon onion powder
- 1 teaspoon dried sage
- ¼ teaspoon chili flakes
- ¼ teaspoon ground black pepper
- 1 tablespoon of sea salt

Directions:

1. Mix mayonnaise and Italian seasoning in a small bowl.
2. Set aside for 30 minutes or more to let the flavors develop.
3. Check if it needs additional seasoning.
4. Keep refrigerated for up to 4-5 days

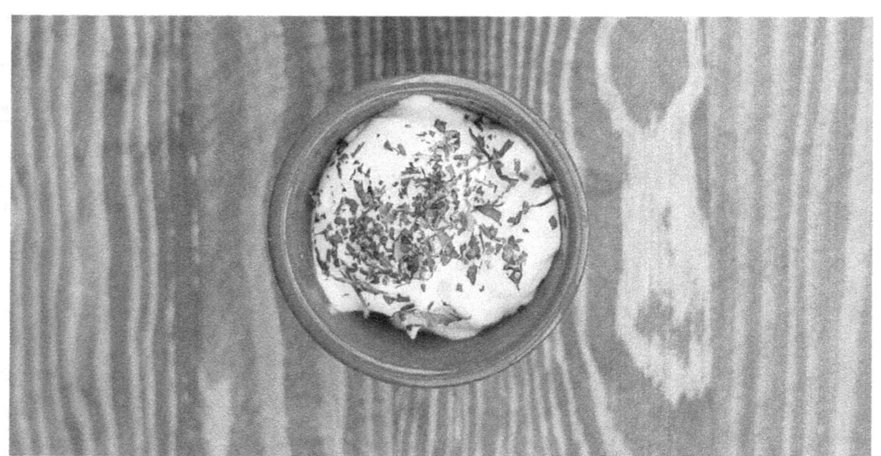

 **30 mins** 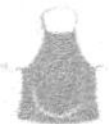 **0 mins** 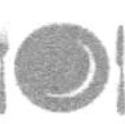 **3/4** 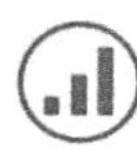 Calories: 61 - Fat: 3g - Fiber: 1,5g
Carbs: 21,4g - Protein: 0g

Chapter 17

Drinks: Juices and Smoothies

GRAPE SMOOTHIE

Ingredients:

- 2 cups red seedless grapes
- ¼ cup (2 fl oz – 60 ml) fruit juice
- ½ cup plain yogurt
- 1 cup ice

Directions:

1. Add fruit juice to the blender. At that time, put in the yogurt and grapes.
2. Add the ice last.
3. Blend until smooth, and enjoy!

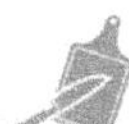 **5 mins** 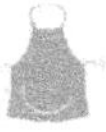 **0 mins** 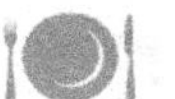 1

Calories: 160 - Fat: 4,1g - Fiber: 1,5g
Carbs: 40g - Protein: 2,5g

BLACK FOREST SMOOTHIE

Ingredients:

- (50 g) or ¼ cup frozen cherries
- 1 handful kale
- 1 Medjool date
- 2 tsp cocoa powder
- 1 tsp chia seeds
- 4 fl oz (120 ml) milk or soya milk

Directions:

1. Place all the ingredients into a blender and process until smooth and creamy.

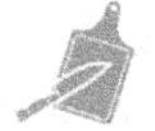 **5 mins** 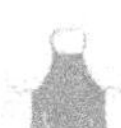 **0 mins**  1 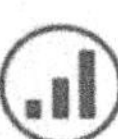

Calories: 145 - Fat: 2,5g - Fiber: 3g
Carbs: 57,9g - Protein: 1g

Ingredients:

- 2 cups lightly packed chopped kale leaves, stems removed
- ¼ cup frozen pineapple pieces
- 1 frozen medium banana, cut into chunks
- ¼ cup non-fat Greek yogurt
- 2 teaspoons honey
- ¾ cup unsweetened vanilla almond milk, or any milk of choice
- 2 tablespoons peanut butter, creamy or crunchy

Directions:

1. Place all the ingredients in a blender.
2. Blend until smooth.
3. Add more milk as needed to reach desired consistency.
4. Enjoy immediately!

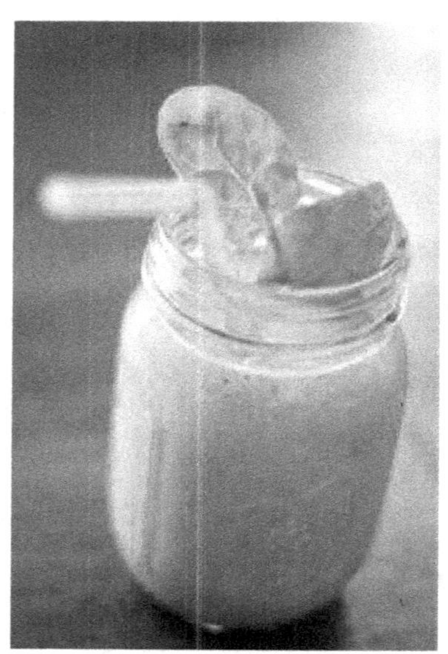

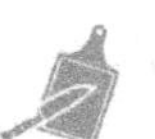 **5/10 mins**

 **0 mins**

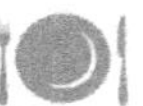 1

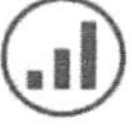 Calories: 187 - Fat: 7,5g - Fiber: 2,6g
Carbs: 14,1g - Protein: 2g

Ingredients:

- 1 cup kale, stalks removed
- 1 teaspoon turmeric
- 1 cup strawberries
- ½ cup of coconut yogurt
- 6 walnut halves
- 1 tablespoon raw cacao powder
- 1-2 mm slice of bird's eye chili
- 1 cup (8 fl oz – 250 ml) unsweetened almond milk
- 1 pitted Medjool date

Directions:

1. Blend together all the ingredients and enjoy immediately!
2. Be careful how much almond milk you add so you can choose the consistency of your favorite.

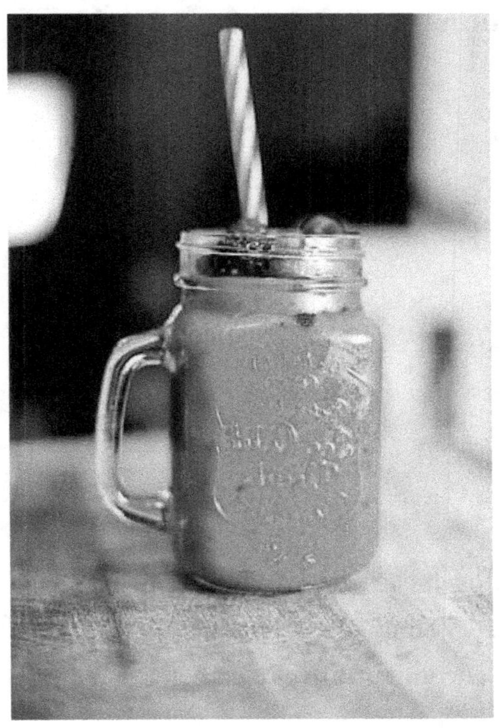

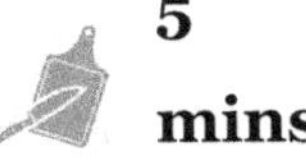 **5 mins**

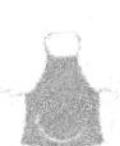 **0 mins**

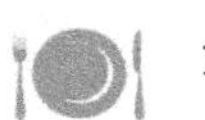 1

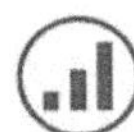 Calories: 176 - Fat: 2,1g - Fiber: 4g
Carbs: 13,5g - Protein: 1g

Ingredients:

- 1 banana
- 2 tsp matcha green tea powder
- ½ tsp vanilla bean (paste or scraped from a vanilla bean pod)
- 1 cup (8fl oz – 250 ml) milk
- 4-5 ice cubes
- 2 tsp honey

Directions:

1. Add all ingredients except the matcha to a blender.
2. Blend until smooth.
3. Sprinkle in the matcha tea powder, stir well or blend a few seconds more (or add cooled green tea).

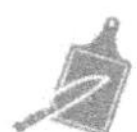 **5 mins**   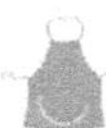 **0 mins**    **1**   (.il) Calories: 118,6 - Fat: 2,1g - Fiber: 4,7g
Carbs: 45g - Protein: 0,8g

APPLE-CUCUMBER JUICE

Ingredients:

- 1 large apple, cored and sliced
- ½ pc large cucumbers, sliced
- 2 celery stalks
- ¼ inch piece fresh ginger, peeled
- ½ lemon, peeled

Directions:

1. Add all ingredients into a juicer and extract the juice.
2. Pour into a glass and serve immediately.
3. Best when apples and cucumbers are chilled before juicing.

 **5/10 mins**    **0 mins**   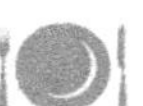 **1**   (.il) Calories: 117,5 - Fat: 2,1g - Fiber: 5,1g
Carbs: 38g - Protein: 0,9g

FRAGRANT TURMERIC TEA

Ingredients:

- 3 teaspoons of ground turmeric
- 1 pc orange, zest only
- 1 tbsp Honey with lemon slices
- 1 tablespoon of freshly grated ginger.

Directions:

1. Put the turmeric, orange zest, and ginger into a teapot filled with the boiling water and allow to infuse with water for up to 5 minutes.
2. Filter with a sieve and pour into serving cups.
3. Add honey and lemon slice as needed.

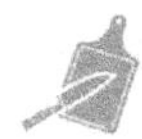 **5 mins**
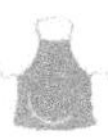 **15 mins**
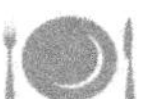 1

Calories: 98 - Fat: 0,5g - Fiber: 3,7g
Carbs: 29,8g - Protein: 1g

THE DAILY GREEN SMOOTHIE

Ingredients:

- Half-peeled, chopped avocado
- 1 large handful parsley
- 1 tablespoon (1/4 fl oz – 10 ml) olive oil
- 1 teaspoon spirulina
- 2 tablespoons of chopped mixed seeds
- ½ fl oz of water – (typically, 120 ml or ½ cup)

Directions:

1. Put all the ingredients together in a blender and blend thoroughly.
2. Serve chilled and enjoy!

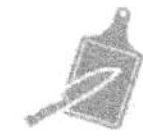 **10 mins**
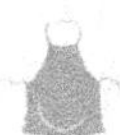 **0 mins**
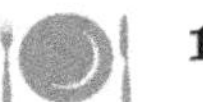 1

Calories: 118 - Fat: 4,8g - Fiber: 6,1g
Carbs: 49,8g - Protein: 7g

Ingredients:

- 1 ½ oz chard
- 1 oz kumquats
- 1 kiwi - peeled
- 1 teaspoon noni fruit powder
- 1 tablespoon quinoa flakes
- 1 cup (8 fl oz – 250 ml) of water

Directions:

1. Put all the ingredients together in a blender and blend thoroughly.
2. Serve chilled and enjoy!

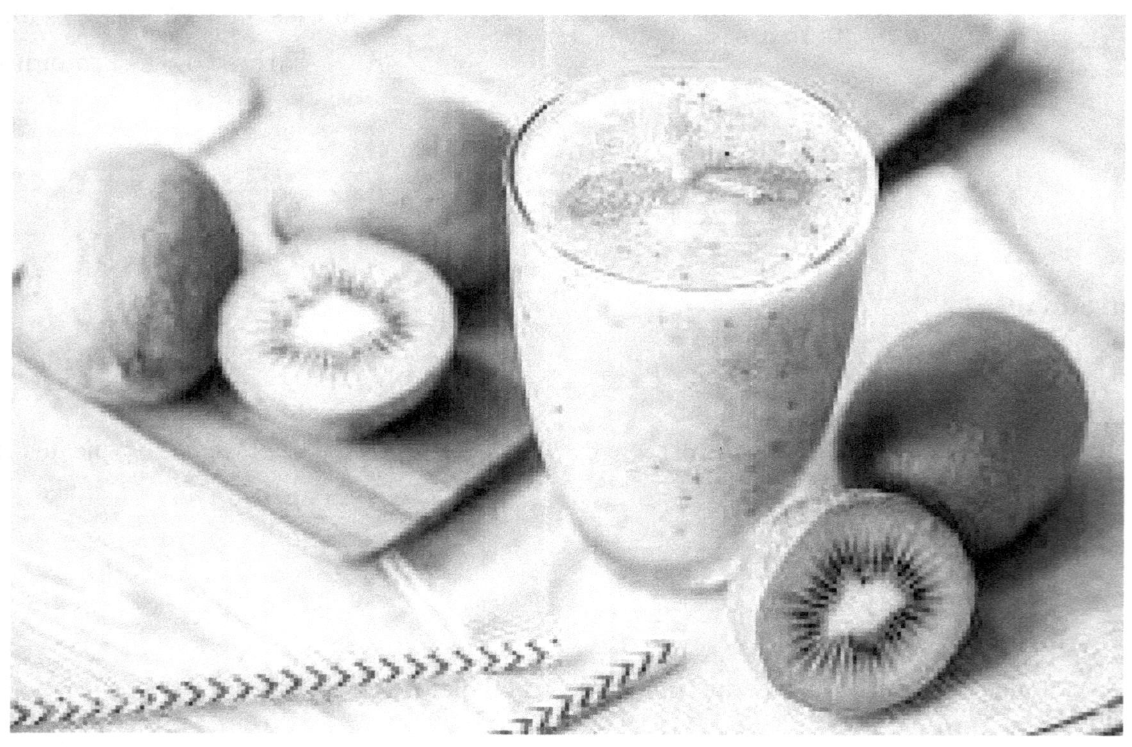

 **5/10 mins**

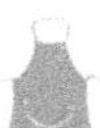 **0 mins**

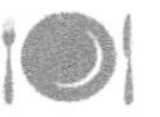 1

Calories: 137,5 - Fat: 1,5g - Fiber: 4,8g
Carbs: 38,5g - Protein: 7g

CELERY SMOOTHIE

Ingredients:

- 2 stalks celery
- 2 cups cabbage
- 2 tbsp (1 fl oz- 30 ml) lemon juice
- 1 tsp dried dill
- ½ tsp juniper berries
- Extra Water – optionally added to dilute the consistency

Directions:

1. Place all ingredients together in a blender and blend thoroughly.
2. Serve chilled and enjoy!

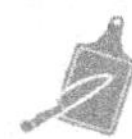 **5 mins**   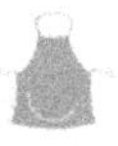 **0 mins**   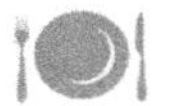 1    Calories: 125,1 - Fat: 1,2g - Fiber: 4,3g
Carbs: 38g - Protein: 3,1g

BERRY BLASTER

Ingredients:

- 1 cup blueberries
- 1 cup cilantro (add more to taste)
- 1 cup raspberries
- 3–4 tablespoons carob powder
- 2 cups (16 fl oz – 500 ml) of fresh orange or tangerine juice
- Extra Water – optionally added to dilute the consistency

Directions:

1. Place all ingredients together in a blender and blend thoroughly.
2. Serve chilled and enjoy!

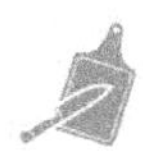 **5 mins**   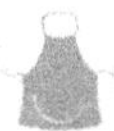 **0 mins**    1    Calories: 120 - Fat: 1,2g - Fiber: 3,7g
Carbs: 35g - Protein: 5g

KALE AND CUCUMBER SMOOTHIE

Ingredients:

- 1 handful kale
- 2-inch cucumber – sliced, chopped
- Half-squeezed lime
- 1 medium mango, peeled & chopped
- 1 tablespoon goji berries
- Extra Water – optionally added to dilute the consistency

Directions:

1. Place all ingredients together in a blender and blend thoroughly.
2. Serve chilled and enjoy!

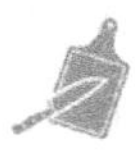 **5 mins**  **0 mins** 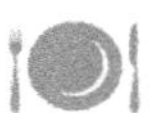 **1**  Calories: 125 - Fat: 1,4g - Fiber: 6g
Carbs: 34g - Protein: 7g

KALE AND BLACK CURRANTS SMOOTHIE

Ingredients:

- 6 ice cubes
- 1 ½ oz (40 g) of blackcurrants, washed and remove stalks
- 1 ripe banana
- 10 baby kale leaves, stalks removed
- 1 cup of freshly made matcha green tea
- 2 tsp of honey

Directions:

1. Dissolve the honey in fresh and warm green tea.
2. Blend together the entire ingredients in a food processor until the mixture is smooth.
3. Serve right away.

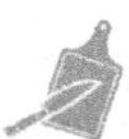 **5 mins** 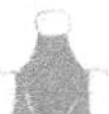 **0 mins**  **1** 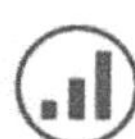 Calories: 85 - Fat: 3g - Fiber: 9g
Carbs: 15g - Protein: 2,5g

GRAPE AND MELON SMOOTHIE

Ingredients:

- 3 ½ oz (100 g) of cantaloupe melon, peeled, seed removed and cut into chunks
- 3 ½ oz (100 g) red seedless grapes
- 1 handful (1 oz - 30 g) of young spinach leaves, stalks removed
- ½ peeled cucumber, seeded and roughly chopped

Directions:

1. Combine together the entire ingredients in a blender until you have a smooth mixture.
2. Serve in a glass.

 **5 mins** 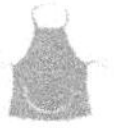 **0 mins** 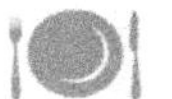 **1**  Calories: 120 - Fat: 2,1g - Fiber: 12,5g
Carbs: 20g - Protein: 3,2g

CHOCOLATE STRAWBERRY MILK

Ingredients:

- 5 ½ oz (150 g) strawberries, hulled and halved
- 1 tbsp cocoa powder (100 % cocoa)
- 2 pcs (1/3 oz) pitted Medjool dates
- 1/3 oz (10 g) walnuts
- 7 fl oz (200 ml) 1milk or dairy-free alternative

Directions:

1. Place all the ingredients in a blender and blitz until smooth.

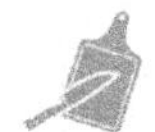 **5 mins** 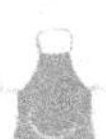 **0 mins** 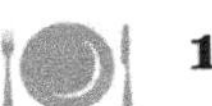 **1** 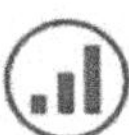 Calories: 141 - Fat: 2,5g - Fiber: 3g
Carbs: 57g - Protein: 5g

Conclusion

There are a thousand and one different diets to lose weight. Every day, a new method to lose weight appears that leaves us homiletics, and that makes us jump on the bandwagon of diets that promise results in a very short time. Although not all of these diets are healthy, there are some that have risen to fame due to the celebrities who have followed it. The last to jump into the fray?

The sirtfood diet that promises to make you lose around three kilos a week, and that seems, Adele has followed to lose 70 kilos.

While half the world is waiting for Adele to release a new album, the other half is obsessed with her weight change. And the rumors are that he would have succeeded with the Sirtfood diet.

This diet began to be a trend since it included the option of including dark chocolate and wine to the nutritional plan. The Sirtfood diet is quite simple and easy to get around since it focuses on foods get from sources of a plant. It encourages fruit, vegetables, whole grains, legumes, seeds, and nuts to eat, which means that most of what you eat is made up of these foods.

You may think it's a vegetarian diet or classic vegan at first. It is not just a diet based on plants; it is flexible considerably and does not boycott milk, seafood, meat, and eggs. It's easy-going and inclusive approach makes this diet attractive—after all, no one likes rules!

Sirtfood also helps preserve muscles, the tissue with the highest energy consumption. Sit-ins activate muscle stem cells. This works on the same principle as strength training: muscles are stressed - here by exertion, in the diet by lack of energy - the repair mechanism starts, new muscle mass is created. More muscle means more energy consumption and is the best remedy for the yo-yo effect.

The Sirtfood Diet is a diet of addition, not isolation, and Sirtfoods are widely accessible and affordable for all. This is a diet that supports you to pick up your sword and fork and enjoy eating delicious fresh food while discussing the health and weight-loss benefits.

You have not only learned the basic information required to start the Sirtfood diet, but you have also gained much more than that! By learning how to meal plan, prep, and storage, you will be able to easily master the Sirt food diet with little day-to-day effort required.

You will be able to enjoy delicious meals at a moment's notice without having to struggle after a long day of work. By just preparing a little ahead of time, you can have a fridge and freezer fully stocked with delicious homemade meals perfectly suited to your taste.

Whether you start out following the Sirt diet to the letter or simply experimenting and enjoying the dishes, you are sure to experience benefits and fall in love with food all over again. What are you waiting for? With just a little effort and time in the kitchen, you can get on your way to success.

Thank you for reading this book! I hope that you find the success you are looking for. If you enjoy the delicious recipes in this book!